RIPPED DAD: FIT AFTER 45

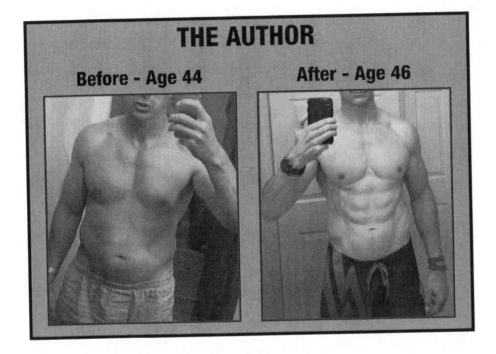

THE AUTHOR

Before - Age 44   After - Age 46

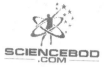

Table of Contents

Introduction 5

1. Mental Preparation: A Long Haul and Not a Short Journey ...6

GET RID OF THE NEGATIVITY 13
LET GO OF MISPERCEPTIONS 15

2. Getting Ripped: Exercise Beyond the Basics 17

THE IMPORTANCE OF LIFTING WEIGHTS...17
HYPERTROPHY AND MUSCLE DEVELOPMENT 22
RESISTANCE TRAINING VARIABLES 25
THE FLOW ZONE 36
CARDIO IN WEIGHT LOSS AND FITNESS 39
HIGH-INTENSITY INTERVAL TRAINING 48
WHAT IS THE IDEAL TRAINING PROGRAM?.....................................51
WHAT TO CONSIDER IN SETTING UP A PLAN....................................55
THE RIPPED DAD 12-WEEK WORKOUT PROGRAM 63
DAD FITNESS OPPORTUNITIES..90
PLATEAUS AND TRACKING PERFORMANCE.......................................93
FITNESS TRACKERS AND OTHER HELPFUL TOOLS...............................97

3. Nutrition And Supplements 103

DIET COMES FIRST 103
PROTEIN...108
DIET OPTIONS 113
THE RIPPED DAD SAMPLE SEVEN-DAY KETOGENIC MEAL PLAN....................115
THE BIG PICTURE 132
SUPPLEMENTS 132

4. Motivation for Lifestyle Changes 146

ANTI-AGING 146
MOTIVATION EVOLUTION 151

Endnotes..156

Introduction

As we walked the teeming streets of Hong Kong in the middle of high summer, the utterly damp heat felt like a weighted vest. Sweat drained from nearly every pore. My drenched shirt clung to my belly and the small of my back revealing to the world around us the contours of my middle-aged body in decline.

To my forty-four-year-old self's horror, my teenage son, taking notice, began loudly chanting, "Daaaaad Bod! Daaaad Bod!" for all to hear. He thought he was hilarious. I thought, "My God, he's right." But the mocking of my son served as the wake-up call I needed.

Today, two years later, at age forty-six, I can honestly say that I am "ripped". I am literally in the best shape of my life. I have a "six-pack" and "guns". My waist measures in at forty-five percent of my height. I keep up with all but the fittest 20-somethings in the gym. Just the other day, a professional bodybuilder at the gym I work out at asked me when I was going to start competing. How did I do it? More importantly, how can you do it?

The answer is contained in this book.

Are you ready to begin your journey? Are you ready to get healthy, fit, and lean? Are you ready improve your vitality and increase the length of your "health-span"? Are you ready to add years to your life? Are you ready to start being noticed and desired again by women? Are you ready to be excited to take your shirt off? Are you ready to get ripped?

1. Mental Preparation: A Long Haul and Not a Short Journey

Making the decision to "get ripped"- to radically improve your "body composition" by increasing muscle mass and melting away stored body fat as a man in midlife is going to present you with challenges. Nothing worthwhile ever comes easy. However, it is more than possible to obtain a ripped physique. Middle-aged men do have the ability to put on muscle and to shed fat.

You may have come to believe that past a certain age, a "dad bod" was just something that happened as you aged. You may have become conditioned to accept that as you entered midlife there was no going back to the body of your youth. You may assume that the bodies of the men you see on the covers of fitness magazines and on late-night exercise equipment infomercials are unachievable fantasies. If so, you are not correct.

You can have six-pack abs. You can have bulging biceps. You can have a sculpted chest. You can improve your health and add years to your life.

What men over the age of 45 must realize is that what used to take a few weeks in the gym to accomplish in their twenties is now going to take a little longer. Why is this?

First, as you age, your levels of testosterone decline. Testosterone has a direct impact on your ability to maintain and build muscle. A 1999 study from the *Journal of Endocrinological Investigation* stated, "testosterone induces muscle cell hypertrophy". "Hypertrophy" is a term we will talk about more in-depth later. For now, however, hypertrophy means bigger muscles. It is the opposite of a term you have probably heard before: "atrophy", which means the shrinking or wasting of muscles. Further, the same study also affirmed that declining testosterone levels with age are correlated with increased fat mass and a decrease in lean body mass. [1]

The second factor is related to the first but encompasses a broader condition called "sarcopenia". As defined in an article from *The Journals of Gerontology*, sarcopenia is "the loss of muscle mass and strength with age". [2] The process of sarcopenia begins in our 30's and accelerates as we age - unless we take steps to fight it. A 2014 study from Germany found, "Muscle strength declines from people aged less than 40 years to those older than 40 years between 16.6% and 40.9%" [3] If we allow sarcopenia to progress unimpeded, by our 70's we risk losing up to fifty percent of our muscle mass. [4]

In a nutshell, sarcopenia is the reason, for example, athletes in their twenties typically outperform older athletes. No big deal, right?

Wrong. Over decades, sarcopenia results in frailty and is a significant driver of mortality as we age. [5] Frailty often results in falls because seniors have lost so much muscle mass and coordination as a result of sarcopenia that they no longer possess the agility and coordination to maintain balance. Falls are the leading cause of death for people 65 and older. Beyond that, falls often indirectly result in death for older individuals. In a study conducted out of Arizona State University, 31% of patients over 60 years old admitted to the hospital for a fall died within three years. [6] Among people age 65 to 69, one in 200 falls results in a hip fracture. After age 85, that figure increases to one in ten. One quarter of older people who fracture their hip will die within six months from the injury. [7]

That is the future most of us face unless we act now to ensure our vitality and extend our lives. Pretty bleak, huh?

Yes, it is. But you have an alternative. You have a say in the matter. You can do something about it.

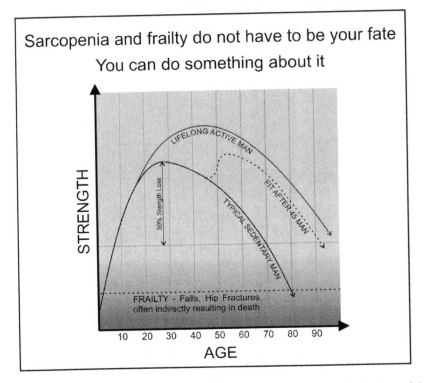

Sarcopenia and frailty do not have to be your fate
You can do something about it

(Figure: Graph of STRENGTH vs AGE showing LIFELONG ACTIVE MAN, FIT AFTER 45 MAN, TYPICAL SEDENTARY MAN curves, 50% Strength Loss marker, and FRAILTY - Falls, Hip Fractures often indirectly resulting in death line. AGE axis marked 10 20 30 40 50 60 70 80 90.)

There is every reason for optimism. Fortunately, getting ripped is the perfect antidote to the looming specter of old age and decline. Science has established beyond a doubt that you can build muscle and decrease body fat – get ripped - well past age 45, and, in fact, into your sixties and beyond.

Do not hesitate to begin. The longer you wait, the more that aging will ravage your body and the more difficult it will be to get the ripped body you want. You need to start now. Do not put it off another day.

As the ancient Chinese philosopher and writer Lao Tzu explains in the *Tao Te Ching*: "The tree you can't reach your arms around grew from a tiny seedling. The nine-story tower rises from a heap of clay. The ten-thousand-mile journey begins beneath your foot." [8]

As a first step, examine the evidence for optimism. A 2001 study published in *The Journal of Applied Physiology* evaluated two groups of men: a group of 46-year-old and a group of 64-year-old men before and after a sixteen-week long exercise regimen. The study found that a "heavy-resistance training program combined with explosive exercises led to large gains in maximal dynamic strength and power-load characteristics." Further, "gains in strength were associated in both groups with considerable muscular hypertrophy." [9] Remember? Hypertrophy equals bigger muscles. That is a good thing.

Another study published in 1999, also from *The Journal of Applied Physiology* examined the effect of a ten-week heavy resistance training program on a group of 62-year-old men. After ten weeks, not only did muscle cross-sectional area increase but the group also "demonstrated a significant increase in total testosterone in response to exercise stress along with significant decreases in resting cortisol." [10]

In simple terms, cortisol is the body's "stress" hormone. A 2013 article from *Psychology Today* described cortisol as "Public Enemy No. 1". The article explained, "Scientists have known for years that elevated cortisol levels: interfere with learning and memory, lower immune function and bone density, increase weight gain, blood pressure, cholesterol, heart disease... The list goes on and on." [11] In most cases, reducing cortisol levels is very desirable.

And the scientific evidence continues: a 2009 study from *The Journal of Strength and Conditioning Research* determined "middle-age men lost significantly more fat mass and significantly decreased percent body fat compared with college-age men" after an eight-week resistance training program. [12]

So, rejoice. Ditch any notion you may have that middle-age for men is equivalent to a dad bod, a beer belly, muffin top, or floppy love handles. That is cultural baggage that has been foisted upon us. It is garbage. As a middle-aged man, you can turn your body into a ripped, continual fat-burning machine.

Results are virtually guaranteed if you take the first step, if you persist, and if you faithfully stick to the principles that, time and again, have been proven by science to result in increased muscle mass and a markedly decreased volume of fat. Three months from now, you will thank yourself for embarking on the journey.

But, you must have a plan. Before talking about nutrition, supplements, workouts and the best exercises to develop the ripped, toned body you want, it is essential to start preparing mentally.

Have you thought about why you want to get ripped? What is your motivation? Have you discovered your "why" with respect to improving your body?

While research has shown that the desire for achieving an aesthetically more appealing body can be a compelling first motivation for beginning a fitness program, it is unlikely to sustain you over the long-term. Remember, if simply wanting to look better were enough, everybody would be walking around with a fit, toned body. The fact is that is simply not the case. Just look around you.

77% of American adults agree with the statement: "Having a good shape and looking good is VERY important for me". [13] Yet nearly 40% of adults in the United States are clinically obese. [14] Why the disconnect?

Why do people abandon fitness programs? Why do people quit going to the gym?

A 1997 study out of the University of Rochester found that while aesthetic motives can be powerful reasons for initiating an exercise regime, "body-related motives are not, on average, sufficient to sustain regular exercise regimens, and thus should not be made the most salient justification for engaging in exercise." [15]

In fact, maintaining too much focus on body-related motivations for working out can set yourself up for failure. One of the reasons that men (and women) fail at attempting to get into shape is they do not see instant results. The University of Rochester study explained it "may be that exercisers who were body-oriented, but who did not see immediate gains in appearance or fitness did not continue" [16]

Think about that for a moment: beginning exercisers quit because they did not see immediate gains? What kinds of rapid gains do you expect to achieve when you are just starting something that is brand new to you? You are a beginner. At first, you are going to be incompetent at lifting weights and working out. Initially, you are going to look foolish (trust me, no one cares but you).

You are going to have failures. You are going to do things wrong. You are going to mess up the diet. You are going to realize you should have done this or that differently. It is all part of the process. It is the nature of learning any new skill. Expect it. Welcome it.

The Japanese martial artist and founder of aikido, Morihei Ueshiba said it very well, "Failure is the key to success; each mistake teaches us something." Likewise, entrepreneur, former US Navy SEAL, and commander of the combat-tested Task Unit Bruiser in Ramadi, Iraq, Jocko Willink explains that one of the keys to his success is to react to all negative developments with one word: "Good." He elaborates, "When things are going bad, there is going to be some good that's going to come from it ... Didn't get the job you wanted? Got injured? Sprained my ankle? Got tapped out? Good. Got beat? Good. You learned. Unexpected problems? Good. We have the opportunity to figure out a solution." [17]

If you keep at it, if you respond to your failures and setbacks with persistence and determination, you will prevail. Slowly but surely, you will begin to succeed. As leadership expert John Maxwell says in his book, *Failing Forward*, "The difference between average people and achieving people is their perception of and response to failure." [18]

And never forget the very wise words of personal development mentor and author of *The Monk Who Sold His Ferrari* series, Robin Sharma: "Every pro was once an amateur. Every expert was once a beginner. So, dream big and start now."

Does it make sense to quit because you are not immediately achieving pro level results when you are starting out as a novice? Absolutely not! Yet, "over 50% of individuals who take part in a fitness program will drop out after the first six months." [19]

The key to lasting success is to shift your focus from immediate results to long-term goals and objectives, with milestones in between to track your fitness progression. A University of Georgia research review revealed, "Active people tend to expect and believe that they receive personal health benefits from exercise". [20] Think about the years you can add to your life. Think about how cancer, heart disease, stroke, diabetes, and Alzheimer's would impact your life and your family's life, and how you can dramatically lower your risk for those diseases and disorders by taking fitness seriously. Think about feeling vital and alive.

A 2018 study from the United Kingdom and published in the journal *Age and Ageing* projects that by 2035 the incidence of diseases and disorders is expected to skyrocket among the older population due to increasing rates of poor health behaviors such as inactivity and obesity. Rates of cancer are forecast to increase by 179.4%, arthritis by 91.6%, dementia by 86.1%, stroke by 84.2%, diabetes by 118.1%, and high blood pressure by 69.5%. Moreover, dramatically more people will be stricken by multiple ailments than today. [21]

Do you want this for your life?

Think about being present and engaged for important events in your children's lives – birthdays, graduations, weddings, and career achievements. Think about having enough energy to one day play with your grandchildren.

Think about enjoying your retirement – exploring distant locales, splashing and swimming in tropical waters, skiing down slopes, and running on lush green grass far past the age when most of your peers have relegated themselves to the sofa in submission to the nagging aches, pains, and conditions that have finally caught up with them after decades of neglecting their bodies.

Overcome your own objections to getting fit. Do whatever you have to do to convince yourself. It is quite literally your own life and well-being that is at stake.

You are reading this book because you have already determined that improving your body composition and losing weight – getting ripped - is important. This book will focus on the science and the information behind building lean muscle and losing weight in the form of fat. The specific workout routines and weights you choose, along with your diet, will be up to you. With this personalized approach, rather than a prescription, you can craft the fitness and lifestyle program that works for your life and allows you to reach your goals.

Get Rid of the Negativity

The first step in getting ready to get ripped is to remove all the negative self-talk you may have with regards to this journey. Many guys start out with a great level of self-confidence and the best of intentions, but the first trip to the gym turns out to also be the last.

Try this experiment: pop into any given gym during the first or second week of January. Then, revisit the same gym on February 10 or later. You will notice a difference. In fact, this ever-so-predictable drop off in gym attendance after the New Year is so notorious, it has its own name: "The Fitness Cliff". In a 2016 article from CBS News, representatives from the Gold's Gym chain explained, "What we see from Gold's Gym's proprietary research is that Tuesday, February 9th is the Fitness Cliff -- the day when New Year's Resolutions go astray, gym check-ins begin to steadily decline and members begin to lose focus on their goals". [22]

This is going to be a change in your routine and your daily life. It is going to mean making some modifications in your schedule. It certainly will mean prioritizing your workout time and developing a greater sense of the choices you are making that are either helping or hindering your progress.

One of your first major priorities will be finding time in your day to work out. While there will be some exercises you can do at home and with the kids, if you really want to develop your muscle and reduce body fat, the gym is where you need to be. This may mean setting up a home gym or arranging care for your children while you hit the fitness center.

A lot of gyms, particularly in larger urban areas, now offer on-site daycare. This can be ideal for dads as young kids can go with you to the gym and have supervised play activities with other kids while you work out, and then you can both do something together afterward. Older and younger kids will benefit from seeing your example of being at the gym and it will help them to incorporate fitness and health into their daily lives from a young age.

Older sons and daughters may also enjoy working out with dad. This is a terrific mentorship and bonding opportunity. It also helps your children to establish their own healthy routines and practices. Of course, for cardio workouts that include jogging,

14

older children may love running with dad, which is another excellent way to spend some quality time. Or they may appreciate the opportunity to ride their bicycle alongside you as you run the path in the park or along the boardwalk. Toddlers may be thrilled to ride in a baby jogger with dad as you go for a run. Be creative.

Let Go of Misperceptions

It is also important as part of getting rid of negativity to lose the misperceptions and myths that you may be holding onto about how to get ripped and how to improve your overall fitness level.

Many of the specifics of these fitness myths will be addressed as they come up in the following sections. It is very likely you have "facts" you think are correct about nutrition during weight loss and muscle building, how long you should work out, the supplements you should take, and even what type of exercises you are doing.

It is important to avoid assuming these "gym truths" are really the facts and become interested in learning the evidence-based science behind turning your body into the lean, toned and ripped body you want. You may be surprised how holding on to these old, outdated ideas about getting fit may be sabotaging your efforts and creating frustration resulting in a lack of progress, possible injury, and maybe worst of all, creating or reinforcing a belief that a ripped body is unachievable for you.

You must educate yourself. Do not rely on what your coach or gym teacher taught you in high school. Do not believe all the "bro science" you picked up from your buddies or from random fitness blogs on the internet. Do not buy into the siren call of the latest easy workout that promises quick results in a few minutes per week on the cover of glossy men's fitness magazines at the checkout aisle.

Please understand "that it takes an average of seventeen years for research evidence to reach clinical practice." [23] That means what you are hearing in terms of fitness recommendations could be seventeen years or more behind the findings of the latest research unless you decide to take responsibility for keeping yourself educated. Google Scholar, PubMed, and Examine.com are examples of three first-rate resources on the internet to keep abreast of the latest scientific information. There are also many excellent YouTube channels and podcasts available offering expert advice and insight on some of the most current thinking in the fitness community. Examples of some of these are Athlean-X and MI40 Muscle Intelligence with Ben Pakulski on YouTube and the podcasts Sigma Nutrition Radio, STEM Talk and Nourish Balance Thrive. These resources offer significant troves of free content. There are many others.

Setting up a plan, understanding your goals, tracking your progress and beginning to educate yourself about the latest fitness science are all parts of the mental preparation for the life-changing journey you are about to embark upon.

2. Getting Ripped: Exercise Beyond the Basics

There are three basic components that you will have to consider when you are designing your fitness plan over the age of 45. These are not random issues, and there is significant scientific study on how to effectively build muscle and lose weight. Unfortunately, scientific studies are not that engaging or entertaining, so watered-down, misinterpreted, out-of-context types of concepts about getting fit tend to continue to thrive.

The three basic components you will need to consider include creating a calorie deficit for weight loss, eating the right foods and supplements for muscle gain, and making the plan sustainable. There are a lot of details in each of these elements, but if you keep it focused on those three issues, you will see weight loss and muscle gain. Keep in mind, the caloric deficit is only to lose fat, once you want to start to build muscle, you will need to eat to fuel the growth of muscle cells, but it will need to be the right types of foods.

The following chapters will focus on eating the appropriate foods and supplements as well as how to stay motivated and focused on your health and well-being, but this chapter is centered around what science and fitness experts know to be the most effective ways for adult males to build muscle and lose weight.

The Importance of Lifting Weights

There is a reason that the gym becomes a central part of any plan for a man over the age of 45: to gain muscle size, strength, tone, and definition. You cannot jog, sprint or interval train

17

yourself into a ripped physique. It takes time engaging in resistance-based exercise to build the muscle fibers and shed fat. Resistance-based exercise most commonly takes the form of lifting weights.

Let's take a closer look at why it is important to hit the gym on a regular basis – at least several times per week. While all forms of exercise are important, and there will be a discussion about cardio and other forms of exercise in getting and staying in shape, there are distinct benefits to resistance-based exercise regimens that are easy to not only see but also to feel almost immediately after starting a routine.

By lifting weights on a regular basis, and using a strategic, educated approach to lifting, your body improves body holistically, developing a stronger frame that helps to protect from age-related decline and injuries later in life. Weight-lifting offers a host of benefits to men, especially as they progress into mid-life. Here is the abstract from a 2012 review published in *Current Sports Medicine Reports* that describes resistance training as "medicine":

> Inactive adults experience a 3% to 8% loss of muscle mass per decade, accompanied by resting metabolic rate reduction and fat accumulation. Ten weeks of resistance training may increase lean weight by 1.4 kg, increase resting metabolic rate by 7%, and reduce fat weight by 1.8 kg. Benefits of resistance training include improved physical performance, movement control, walking speed, functional independence, cognitive abilities, and self-esteem. Resistance training may assist prevention and management of type 2 diabetes by decreasing visceral fat, reducing HbA1c, increasing the density of glucose transporter type 4, and improving insulin sensitivity. Resistance training may enhance cardiovascular health, by reducing resting blood pressure, decreasing low-density lipoprotein cholesterol and triglycerides, and increasing high-density lipoprotein cholesterol. Resistance

training may promote bone development, with studies showing 1% to 3% increase in bone mineral density. Resistance training may be effective for reducing low back pain and easing discomfort associated with arthritis and fibromyalgia and has been shown to reverse specific aging factors in skeletal muscle. [24]

Regular weight lifting will improve posture and boost natural production of testosterone. Additionally, it helps to reduce stress hormones in the body, promoting a calmer sense of well-being while helping to reduce anxiety and stress. Lower levels of stress hormones, particularly cortisol, also help to prevent the body from storing fat, which occurs as a natural response to chronic stress. Men that routinely lift weights tend to be sounder and better sleepers, which has a wide range of health implications, including better immune responses and increased weight loss.

Finally, and this is critical, lifting weights burns fat faster over a period of weeks and months than other forms of exercise. Why? The major reason is that resistance training builds muscle. As lean muscle burns more calories than fat, it serves to keep your weight maintained once you reach your goal. Of course, once you see results, you will also be motivated to stay on track with your new healthy lifestyle. Do you really want to destroy your gains and sidetrack your progress by eating that ice cream or scarfing down that bag of chips?

Echoing the same principle cited in the above research review regarding resistance training as "medicine", an article in the British newspaper, *The Telegraph* entitled "Why Lifting Is The New Running For The Over-40's", underlined the importance of resistance training as men enter into their forties by explaining what happens in the absence of a strength training program: "Each decade after thirty, muscle declines by 3-8 per cent and because it has a higher metabolic rate than fat, the more muscle you have, the more calories you burn not only during exercise but also at rest." If you do not battle against this natural tendency to lose muscle mass as the years progress with resistance training, your body composition will shift more and more toward fat. As that cycle progresses, you enter into a kind of death sprial: more fat equals a slower metabolism which leads to more fat and an even slower metabolism. [25]

This is where the term "middle-age spread" really starts to hit home. The lifestyle that may have kept you lean in your twenties and thirties simply is not effective anymore. Your body is actually now less efficient, so there has to be compensation in the form of eating healthier and reducing caloric intake combined with muscle-building exercises..

In fact, according to the article from *The Telegraph*, by adding between two and four pounds of muscle to the body you will burn an additional one hundred calories per day, just in your resting state. When weightlifting and cardiovascular training is added to your routine, it is possible to continue to cut fat, add muscle and increase the metabolic rate. This will not only help with shedding pounds, but it will also help to prevent future weight gain while adding lean, efficient muscle mass.

When you first start going to the gym, the initial goal behind lifting weights is not to immediately start building ripped muscles. That will happen. But you first must learn the proper form and method of lifting weights.

According to professional strength coach, former Major League baseball physical therapist, author, and lecturer Jeff Cavaliere, founder of the highly esteemed Athlean-X Training System, it is critical to focus on the movement of the weight and the contraction of the muscle, and not on completing so many repetitions in so many sets with a specific weight. He spells out, "make sure that no matter what exercise you're doing or what primary muscle group you're training that you move EVERY REP of EVERY EXERCISE by C-O-N-T-R-A-C-T-I-N-G the muscle responsible for the movement or exercise". [26]

When you are a beginner at the gym, Mr. Caveliere recommends starting with light weights because initially your objective is, as he explains, to "learn the movement pattern – groove that pattern." He warns that if you skip this step, "you're not only not growing as much as you can because you're not optimally stimulating the muscles you're trying to work but you're setting up bad patterns to just carry over into more shit workouts down the road." [27] Too many amateurs and "gym bros" rely on momentum and bad form to push through to complete a specific number of lifts. Do not be like them.

It is imperative that you understand this point: your goal is absolutely not to go to the gym and repeatedly move a given amount of weight a certain amount of times through a series of exercises so that you can check a box signifying in your mind that "I worked out today". Your goal is not to impress yourself or others with how much weight you lifted regardless of how bad your form is. In the gym, as in much of life, your ego is your enemy. One of India's most respected spiritual leaders, Radhanath Swami put it well in his book *The Journey Home*: "whenever you feed your ego ... you will not succeed." [28]

The objective of resistance exercise is to "feel the burn" by employing movements that have been proven to provide maximally effective contraction throughout a range of motion for the muscle or muscle group you are targeting. You may not think it looks impressive to lighten your load and focus on disciplined form and muscular contraction, but this is the path to success.

It does not matter how loud you grunt nor how much weight you bench press with your back arched up in the air nor how many pullups you do swinging your body up to the bar almost entirely with momentum. What matters is focused contraction of the intended muscle providing the utmost stimulation to the muscle fibers. This is a far more effective method for providing a growth signal to the muscle fibers on a microscopic level than going to the gym and doing X number of sets of eight to twelve repetitions without intensity, or without strict form, or relying on momentum or the recruitment of non-targeted muscle groups to assist. If you fail to make this a focus, you are only cheating yourself and slowing down or killing your gains. Focused contraction of each and every repetition provides much faster results and a vastly more effective way to spend your time in the gym. This is the quickest path toward achieving the ripped body you want. Do not take shortcuts.

Hypertrophy and Muscle Development

We talked a little about "hypertrophy" earlier. We will get into it a little bit deeper here.

Depending on how you count and who you ask, there are anywhere from 650 to 840 named skeletal muscles in the human body. "The dissension comes from those that count the muscles within a complex muscle. For example, the biceps brachii is a complex muscle that has two heads and two different origins however, they insert on the radial tuberosity. Do you count this as one muscle or two?" [29]

Muscles, at their fundamental level, are comprised of muscle fibers. A muscle fiber is a single cell that can vary in length from less than one millimeter to several centimeters. [30] Another name for a single muscle fiber cell is "myofiber". [31] "An individual skeletal muscle may be made up of hundreds, or even thousands, of muscle fibers bundled together and wrapped in a connective tissue covering." [32]

At the muscle fiber level, there are some important distinctions. There are different types of muscle fiber. You have probably heard of the terms "slow twitch" and "fast twitch" muscles. Gaining prominence in the discussion around muscle fibers in the last decade is talking about muscle fibers in terms of "Type I", and "Type II (A and B)" fibers. That can get confusing. However, in reality, it is pretty easy to understand.

"Slow twitch" muscles correspond to muscles comprised primarily of "Type I" muscle fibers. Type I fibers "contract slower, are very durable, and have a high resistance to fatigue. Slow twitch muscle fibers play a role in maintaining posture and are predominantly responsible for lower-intensity activities such as jogging." [33]

"Fast twitch" muscles, conversely, correspond to muscles comprised primarily of "Type II" fibers. Type II fibers are characterized by high power output and low endurance. Within the general classification of Type II fibers, there are two forms: Type II-A and Type II-B. "[Type II-A] fibers have a moderate resistance to fatigue and represent a transition between the two extremes of the [Type I] and [Type II-B] fibers ... Functionally, they are used for prolonged anaerobic activities with a relatively high force output, such as racing 400 meters." Type II-B fibers, "on the other hand, are very sensitive to fatigue and are used for short anaerobic, high force production activities, such as sprinting, hurdling, jumping, and putting the shot. These fibers are also capable of producing more power than [Type I] fibers." [34]

Muscle fiber types vary among different kinds of athletes: "The largest percentage of Type I fibres was found in long distance runners; the smallest in those performing karate and triple jump. The largest percentage of Type IIA fibres was found in swimmers and the smallest in footballers. The largest percentages of Type IIB ... were found in footballers." [35]

"Resistance exercise leads to the preferential hypertrophy of type II fibers." [36] Type I fibers, on the other hand, do not demonstrate a marked hypertrophic response to exercise. [37] Type II muscles fibers are larger and produce more specific force than Type I fibers, and "Type II fibers show greater plasticity in size when compared to Type I fibers, in response to various mechanical stimuli." [38]

Bottom line: Type II fibers grow more in response to resistance exercise. Type I fibers exhibit very little growth. Type II fibers are going to provide you with the vast majority of the growth portion of getting ripped.

What determines your own personal proportion of Type I vs Type II muscle fibers? Recent research has discovered that, "The fiber type composition of a muscle, once thought to be genetically determined, is highly plastic and can be altered in response to functional demands", like lifting weights. [39] That is important because it means you cannot rely on cop-outs like "I do not have a weightlifter's body type" or "it's just not in my genes".

Resistance exercise promotes a sort of virtuous fitness cycle in terms of getting ripped and staving off the age-related ravages of sarcopenia: as your Type II fibers hypertrophy, you signal your body to create a greater proportion of Type II fibers which results in even greater hypertrophy. It is like the famous saying from the Christian scriptures: "... to the one who has, more will be given". [40]

What causes Type II fibers to hypertrophy? "Mechanical overload of skeletal muscle promotes an increase in myofiber cross-sectional area ... Resistance-based exercise provides the optimal 'anabolic' signal to stimulate the protein synthetic response, with increases in muscle protein synthesis ... underlying the growth in individual muscle fibers and total muscle cross-sectional area". [41] What does that mean? It means resistance-based exercise is what causes Type II fibers to grow. Resistance-based exercise causes hypertrophy. Getting ripped is not going to happen without hypertrophy.

As an important aside, it is significant to note that science has not definitively determined exactly what mechanism at the cellular level causes muscles to grow. Scientists know that resistance exercise provides the stimulus for hypertrophy but they are still unsure exactly how that occurs.

Many of us have heard repeatedly over the years that we want to "tear down the muscle fibers". This is called the "muscle damage" hypothesis of muscle hypertrophy. There is, however, no direct, linear correlation between muscle damage and muscle hypertrophy. [42] The mechanism of hypertrophy is extremely complicated. Science has been hard at work for decades attempting to divine the exact processes at work behind hypertrophy. Progress has been made but the ultimate answer has proven elusive. It is likely that the dose-response curve of tearing down the muscle fibers to hypertrophy approximates a bell-shaped curve: some damage to the muscle fiber probably does create a hypertrophic response but too much damage proves counter-productive. What is known for certain is that resistance training is essential to hypertrophy.

Without resistance training, you can go to the gym, work out on the treadmill or elliptical or stationary bike or whatever and get lean, but not get ripped. To add muscle mass and definition, hypertrophy through some form of resistance exercise has to occur.

Resistance Training Variables

When you engage in resistance training, there are many ways to go about it. Can I get ripped if I only work out two days per week? How long should I stay at the gym? Is it best to lift heavy or light? Should I rest for 30 seconds in between sets or for three minutes? What works better: 20 sets or five sets? How fast should I push out my repetitions?

There are many variables at play in a resistance training workout. In this section, we will examine some of the most important variables. As with most questions health-related, the answers will vary depending on the context and your specific situation.

Frequency

The United States Centers for Disease Control recommends that adults engage in some sort of resistance training at least two days per week that works all major muscle groups. [43]

In contrast, a 2016 review study from the journal *Sports Medicine* led by the internationally renowned fitness expert Dr. Brad Schoenfeld stated, "the current body of evidence indicates that frequencies of training twice a week promote superior hypertrophic outcomes to once a week. It can therefore be inferred that the major muscle groups should be trained at least twice a week to maximize muscle growth; whether training a muscle group three times per week is superior to a twice-per-week protocol remains to be determined." [44]

Please notice that this study does not indicate that you should limit your gym visits to two days per week. It is very difficult, if not impossible, to train all the major muscle groups in one workout and maintain the kind of intensity required to produce hypertrophy. No, what this study indicates is that you should train, for example, legs (a major muscle group) two days per week and back (another major muscle group) on a different two days per week than you train legs. Successful, experienced weight lifters group their major muscle group workouts differently but very few, if any, will limit their gym visits to only two days per week.

In 2009, the American College of Sports Medicine published their position stand on resistance training frequency: "The recommendation for training frequency is 2-3 [days per week] for novice training, 3-4 [days per week] for intermediate training, and 4-5 [days per week] for advanced training". [45]

An older study from 2000 published in *The Journal of Strength and Conditioning Research*, compared recreational weightlifters working out one day per week versus three days per week: "The findings suggest that a higher frequency of resistance training, even when volume is held constant, produces superior gains in one-rep-max. However, training only 1 day per week was an effective means of increasing strength, even in experienced recreational weight trainers. From a dose-response perspective, with the total volume of exercise held constant, spreading the training frequency to 3 doses per week produced superior results." [46]

In other words, some training is better than no training but three days per week is better than one day per week. The study did not evaluate the effects of working out more than three days per week. Personally, from my own n = 1, anecdotal perspective, I usually find that lifting weights about five days per week is my own sweet spot. My anecdotal experience is backed up with research from 1982 published in *The Journal of Sports Medicine and Physical Fitness* that found, "Significantly greater muscular strength improvement was observed in the group that trained 5 days per week than groups training with fewer frequencies per week. Sequential strength improvements resulted from increased frequency of training. It was concluded that the more frequent the stress the greater the adaptation." [47] Some weeks I will go to the gym six days. On occasion, I may only make it four days in a week, but that is rare. I am not doing the same workout each time I go to the gym. I end up hitting my major muscle groups about twice per week, sometimes three times per week.

Length of Workout

Much debate surrounds the amount of time that should be spent at the gym for a workout. It seems that there is somewhat of a consensus that has settled upon forty-five minutes to one hour of resistance training to accommodate a good workout. That does not include any time you opt to spend on cardio training after your resistance training session. It also does not include time allotted for warm-up, stretching, or cool-down.

This period of time assumes that you are actively engaged in resistance training during that time period. Time spent socializing, checking your phone, configuring equipment, or day-dreaming will significantly detract from the gains you can achieve and does not count toward time spent working out.

Forty-five minutes to one hour also provides a good test as to whether or not you have worked out with enough intensity during that time period. If you are not exhausted at the end of that period, you probably have not worked out intensely enough. A 2010 review article in the *Journal of Strength and Conditioning Research* stated, "it has been proposed that intense workouts should not last longer than one hour to ensure maximal training capacity throughout the session". [48]

A 2000 study from the *Strength and Conditioning Journal* expanded on that principle by stating, "Long training sessions have been associated with decreased intensity of effort, decreased levels of motivation, and even changes in immune response." [49]

Well-known fitness guru Jason Ferrugia also endorses the forty-five minute to one hour period of time for a workout: "When you start training your body will naturally boost testosterone levels significantly higher than normal. This increased output peaks somewhere around a half hour into your workout. By taking blood samples of their athletes, Eastern Bloc researchers determined that at the 45-minute mark your testosterone levels are coming back down to baseline. And after sixty minutes your body will start to produce less testosterone and more cortisol, which is a hormone that eats muscle tissue and increases body fat storage." [50]

Load and Number of Repetitions

This is another subject upon which there is much debate within the fitness community. Load (heavy or light) is correlated with number of repetitions. In other words, heavy sets are almost always going to be low repetition sets and light sets will typically be high repetition sets. Some fitness experts advocate heavy weight, low repetition workouts while others call for light weight, high repetition workouts. Who is correct?

A 2008 study from the *Journal of Applied Physiology* determined, "light load resistance training was inferior to high load training in evoking adaptive changes in muscle size and contractile strength and was insufficient to induce changes" in muscle size. [51] Whether or not a set is heavy or light is determined by reference to the "one-rep-max" (1RM) weight that the individual is able to lift.

The strength training textbook *Designing Resistance Training Programs* states, "The minimal intensity that can be used to perform a set to momentary voluntary fatigue in young, healthy people to result in increased strength is 60 to 65% of 1RM ... However, progression with resistances in the 50 to 60% of 1RM range may be effective and may result in greater 1RM increases than the use of heavier resistances in some populations (e.g., in children and senior women) ... Additionally, approximately 80% of 1RM results in optimal maximal strength gains in weight-trained people."

This evidence provides us with some useful guidelines in terms of knowing how much load to begin with and how much load to shoot for as we progress in the gym. If you are a complete novice and have little experience lifting weights, swallow your pride and start with the loads recommended for children and women (50-60% of 1RM). A 2013 study in the *Sports Medicine* journal affirms that this is a good way to start as a beginner: "low-load training can increase muscle mass in untrained

29

subjects. Therefore, low-load training to failure appears to be an effective strategy to increase muscle mass during early-stage training." [52] If you have some experience and you are in moderately good shape already, start in the 60-65% 1RM max range. As you improve, aim to ratchet your loads up to the 80% 1RM level.

The American College of Sports Medicine recommends increasing weight by two to ten percent when training at a specific RM load (5RM, 10RM, 12RM, etc.) "when the individual can perform the current workload for one to two repetitions over the desired number". [53]

What about the number of repetitions? In terms of getting ripped, the evidence points toward a moderate number of repetitions. "Repetitions can be classified into 3 basic ranges: low (1-5), moderate (6-12), and high (15+) ... Whether low repetitions or moderate reps evoke a greater hypertrophic response has been a matter of debate, and both produce significant gains in muscle growth. However, there is a prevailing belief that a moderate range of approximately 6-12 repetitions optimizes the hypertrophic response." [54]

Number of repetitions bears some relationship to load via a concept called "time under tension" (TUT). Time under tension is the time that the muscle is engaged during the lift. As mentioned earlier, when slowing down the repetitions you will complete fewer repetitions in the same amount of time, but the time under tension will be increased as the muscles are engaged for a longer period of time on each repetition.

According to Ben Pakulski, IFBB professional bodybuilder, author, coach, podcaster, Mr. Canada winner, and second place finisher at the Arnold Classic, "When the goal is to maximize hypertrophy, always execute an exercise in a manner which allows for maximum continuous tension in the target muscle(s), through a full range of motion, for a total of 40 to 70 seconds, pushing to achieve frequent progressive tension overload!" He emphasizes that this means no resting, pausing or dissipating tension at the top or bottom of a repetition. For sets of 40 seconds duration, he will use heavier weights. For sets of 70 seconds duration, he will use lighter weights. [55]

Using a combination of long-duration sets and lower-duration sets serves to address the varying characteristics of Type I and Type II muscle fibers. Remember from the discussion of muscle fibers, Type I fibers are fatigue- and hypertrophy- resistant. However, they can grow. A 2015 article by Dr. Brad Schoenfeld posted on the *T-Nation* web site explained: "By nature, slow-twitch type I fibers are fatigue-resistant (as opposed to type II fibers, which can produce high levels of force but fatigue rather easily). It therefore stands to reason that you'd need to keep the type I fibers under tension for extended periods to elicit their maximal growth. Short durations with heavy loads simply won't provide enough of a stimulus for fatigue. So, the use of light loads for long TUTs would seem necessary to fully develop the indefatigable slow twitch muscle fibers. Emerging research out of Russia shows that this indeed is the case, with light-load protocols involving high TUTs (50% 1RM) showing more type 1 fiber growth and heavier-loads with lower TUTs (80% 1RM) displaying greater hypertrophy of type II fibers." [56]

In a separate piece featured on *FlexOnline*, Mr. Pakulski explains, in order for hypertrophy to occur, when considering an exercise to incorporate into your workout, you must ask yourself, "Does it create maximum and continuous tension, and does it take a muscle through a full range of motion. As you've all heard before: Muscles don't know how much weight you're lifting, they only know TENSION. A question I'm always asking myself is: How do I create greater tension?" [57]

Realize that the science surrounding TUT is still developing. Some studies conflict with each other. In an article by Dr. Jacob Wilson, CEO of the Applied Science and Performance Institute at Florida State University, which included reporting from several studies, it was found that increasing TUT did not significantly enhance muscle growth, but did increase strength. [58]

Another study from 2012 published in *The Journal of Physiology* found that men performing a leg extension exercise at 30% 1RM with a tempo of six seconds up and six seconds down saw better results in muscle growth than the same exercise performed rapidly at a tempo of one second up and one second down. The researchers concluded in that case, "the time the muscle is under tension during exercise may be important in optimizing muscle growth." [59]

One last thing to consider before wrapping up this section is the idea of training to failure: should you or should you not? A 2018 study from *The Journal of Strength and Conditioning Research* found that sets taken to a point just prior to failure ("volitional interruption") were just as effective as sets taken to failure. [60] Given that going to failure significantly impairs performance ability in subsequent sets thereby reducing training volume, my recommendation is to leave one or two repetitions "in the tank", except perhaps on the last set of an exercise.

It seems that the best interpretation of the current science is that, in general, limit the resistance training portion of your workout to one hour of intense effort employing sets of 6-12 at 40 to 70 seconds per set with an emphasis on the sets around 40 seconds in duration. However, always remember that every human body is different. There are myriad important genetic and environmental variables at play at any given moment. Listen to your body. But always push yourself.

The key is to increase intensity and duration over time. The more that muscles grow, the more they can sustain activity and allow for increased weight, increased repetitions and increased sets. This translates to increased volume and, at the same time, increased time under tension due to the increased repetitions. Volume, by the way, is defined as the number of repetitions times the weight lifted. In other words, dead-lifting 200 pounds ten times yields a volume of 2000 pounds. As you can see, volume is directly correlated to the number of repetitions and weight lifted during a workout. The result of all of this is increased muscle growth and, just as importantly, the ability to turn your body into a fat burning machine, helping to boost both active and resting metabolism for weight loss and effective weight management.

Rest Period Between Sets

The amount of time to spend between sets varies depending on your goal. Since our goal is hypertrophy, we want to select the ideal rest period to maximize muscle growth.

The research surrounding rest periods during a workout session suggests a period of one minute between sets might be ideal. In 2005, the journal *Sports Medicine* pronounced: "If the programme is designed for muscular hypertrophy, shorter rest periods of 1–2 minutes are prescribed". [61] This meshes with the findings of an earlier 1990 study that revealed, using rest periods of one minute between sets at 10RM during a full-body workout consisting of three sets per exercise, produced a "dramatic stimulus to serum hGH (human growth hormone) responses". Compared to a workout using sets at 5RM and three-minute rest periods between sets with three to five sets per exercise, hGH levels nearly doubled in men during the workout with the shorter one-minute rest periods, more than quadrupled for up to fifteen minutes post-workout and then remained approximately double for up to an hour post-workout. [62] 5RM and 10RM is simply a form of terminology used by researchers and experienced weightlifters meaning the heaviest weight you can lift for five repetitions (5RM) or for ten repetitions (10RM) or fifteen repetitions (15RM) or whatever.

Tempo

Tempo refers to the speed at which an individual repetition of an exercise is performed. How fast or how slow should you go. We have already discussed this idea indirectly when we reviewed concepts related to time under tension (TUT). However, it is appropriate to address tempo more directly as a separate piece of the resistance training puzzle as well.

One thing is certain: you do not want to be that guy in the gym attempting to whip through his repetitions with utmost speed – and sometimes accompanied by obnoxious grunts. Those guys are clearly amateurs. They might think the speed with which they perform an exercise is a mark of machismo or strength, but it only serves to clearly identify them as uninformed. Worse, they are setting themselves or even someone else nearby them in the gym for an injury.

Onto the science. Previously, in our discussion of TUT, we discussed how we want our set duration between 40 and 70 seconds, with most sets nearer 40 seconds than 70 seconds to provide the most hypertrophy to our Type II muscle fibers. In our discussion of number of repetitions, we also discovered how a moderate number of repetitions produces the best hypertrophic effect. We defined a moderate number of repetitions as six to twelve. With all of that in mind, if we performed a set of bicep dumbbell curls at 10RM with a duration of 50 seconds, ideally each repetition would last five seconds (50 seconds divided by 10 repetitions = five seconds per repetition).

So, we would shoot for five seconds per repetition. That, however, only partially answers the question of the tempo we would like to aim for during the set. Should we explode quickly during the concentric portion of the repetition? The concentric portion of a repetition, by the way, is the muscle-shortening segment of it. In the case of a bicep dumbbell curl, for example, the concentric portion occurs while you draw the weight toward your body. This is also called the "positive" part of the repetition. Or should you try to draw the concentric portion out for, say, four seconds, and then drop the weight quickly in one second during the eccentric portion (muscle-lengthening portion) of the repetition? The eccentric part of a repetition is also called the "negative". Or, alternatively, should both the concentric and eccentric segments be only one second each – and the isometric portion three seconds? The isometric portion is technically the point at which the muscle is at maximum contraction – the squeeze at the top of the bicep curl, for example. However, in terms of discussing tempo, the isometric portion is more often thought of as the pause between concentric and eccentric portions.

So many variables! Do not fear. Science has also investigated this. For hypertrophy, one study found that the tempo we should aim for is 2:1:2. [63] What does that mean? Tempo numbers are expressed in terms of the eccentric portion first, the isometric portion next, and the concentric portion last. So, for a five-second repetition of the bicep dumbbell curl, we would start by extending the weight from a contracted position and lowering it to the fully extended position in two seconds, pausing for one second, and then raising the dumbbell to the fully contracted position in two seconds, pausing one second, and so on until ten repetitions are completed.

The National Strength and Conditioning Association recommends a tempo for hypertrophy of one to two seconds for the eccentric portion, one second for the isometric phase, and one to two seconds for the concentric portion of the repetition. [64] Ben Pakulski also has practical advice to offer about lifting tempo. He asserts, "If your goal is to constantly be building muscle, you must vary tempo often. This is one of the best-known ways to recruit different muscle fiber types (IA, IIA, IIB). It is advantageous to change the rep tempo of your workouts every 3-6 weeks. Some great examples for hypertrophy are 4010, 6010, 4111, 4021." [65] Notice that Mr. Pakulski uses four numbers, as opposed to three, to describe his tempo scheme.

This format is commonly used by weightlifters to describe their tempos. In the case of "4010": "4" is the eccentric, or "negative" portion of the repetition, "0" is the pause at the bottom before initiating the concentric or "positive" portion of the movement, "1" is the speed of the concentric portion, and the final "0" is the pause in the fully contracted portion at the top of the movement.

The Flow Zone

It is important to realize that there is another factor to consider as well. That factor is critical to maximizing your workout with both weight training as well as with your cardio workout. It is the "X" factor of working out and getting ripped. It is achieving victory in the "inner game". This "inner game" is described in W. Timothy Gallwey's classic *The Inner Game of Tennis* as, "the game that takes place in the mind of the player, and it is played against such obstacles as lapses in concentration, nervousness, self-doubt and self-condemnation. In short, it is played to overcome all habits of mind which inhibit excellence in performance." [66]

As expressed in the book *In The Zone: Transcendent Experience in Sports*, "The ability to call up extraordinary reserves of energy … is a key to outstanding athletic performance", [67] and seems to be preferentially available to those who can access a state of flow.

Getting on top of your own inner game allows you to enter a state of "flow" or "optimal experience", which "results in greater power and accuracy." [68] The Russian world-record setting weightlifter Yuri Vlasov, who won a gold medal for the Soviet Union at the 1960 Olympic Games in Rome described the state of flow like this: "At the peak of tremendous and victorious effort while the blood is pounding in your head, all suddenly becomes quiet within you. Everything seems clearer and whiter than ever

36

before, as if great spotlights had been turned on ... At that moment you have the conviction that you contain all the power in the world, that you are capable of everything ..." [69]

In his book *Flow: The Psychology of Optimal Experience*, Claremont University psychology professor Mihaly Csikszentmihalyi explains how optimal experiences are usually not relaxing and easy experiences:

> The best moments usually occur if a person's body or mind is stretched to its limits in a voluntary effort to accomplish something difficult and worthwhile. Optimal experience is thus something that we make happen. For a child, it could be placing with trembling fingers the last block on a tower she has built, higher than any she has built so far; for a swimmer, it could be trying to beat his own record ... Such experiences are not necessarily pleasant at the time they occur. The swimmer's muscles might have ached during his most memorable race, his lungs might have felt like exploding, and he might have been dizzy with fatigue – yet these could have been the best moments of his life. Getting control of life is never easy, and sometimes it can be definitely painful. But in the long run optimal experiences add up to a sense of mastery – or perhaps better, a sense of *participation*, in determining the content of life – that comes as close to what is usually meant as happiness as anything else we can conceivably imagine. [70]

Getting into the gym and working on getting your body ripped can provide a perfect vehicle for you to encounter flow and optimal experience as you struggle with your physical, emotional, and spiritual weaknesses, delight in your strengths, and exalt in your victories over self and previous limitations. If you are doing it right, I promise you that there will be much momentary unpleasantness on the path to getting fit – your muscles will ache, your lungs will feel like they are going to explode, and you will be dizzy with fatigue – but there will also be the incomparable reward of becoming one with the moment as you wrestle with all that has held you back and as you push through previous boundaries.

In addition to the physical discomfort, your mind will also lie, cheat, and deceive in its efforts to remain in comfort. There are many days when it seems like I would prefer to stay home, to take it easy, or to watch a movie on Amazon or NetFlix. Warm, fuzzy thoughts of a cozy nap tempt me. I hear myself rationalize, "Just one day off won't matter." On those days, I wage psychological warfare against that part of my brain that prefers comfort. I remember that if I succumb to that inner weakness, I will get the results that go along with weakness. I tell myself, in the words of legendary American pro football player Jerry Rice, "NO!", "Today, I will do what others won't, so tomorrow I can accomplish what others can't."

Mr. Gallwey explains, "Getting the clearest possible image of your desired outcomes is a most useful method" for entering into the state of flow." [71] Incorporating a meditation or visualization practice into your life can be helpful in enabling yourself to clearly envision your goals as reality. Personally, I do both meditation and visualization. There are many apps (Headspace is an outstanding one) available that provide guided meditations. There are YouTube videos that do the same. Most communities have organizations or groups that offer instruction in meditation and group meditations. Another technique I use to help myself more clearly see my goals is a vision board gallery of photos on my phone that I can scroll through during spare moments.

I have also found music to be very helpful for getting me into "the zone". I rarely ever go to the gym without music and a pair of headphones on. A 2018 experiment sponsored by Texas Tech University Health Sciences agreed with this observation, noting, "Music can have a powerful impact on our mood, signaling the brain to release feel-good and energy-boosting chemicals." The experimenters found that subjects in the experiment were able to exercise "significantly longer in the music group compared with the control group." [72]

My taste in music is ever-changing. What motivates me one week loses its touch the next week. And since musical tastes are so personal, I will not recommend any kind of specific music. However, music works very well for me and many others. Consider it as an aid toward getting yourself into the zone.

Ultimately, apps, YouTube videos and music are only props and crutches. Getting into flow and achieving optimal experiences in the zone - getting into a sort of "beast mode" - require you to know with certainty what you are going after and committing your whole heart and spirit to getting after it. That is the land where dragons are slayed, and princesses are rescued: where magic happens. In that zone, the gym becomes not a big room with some equipment in it but instead transforms into a proving ground of sorts – a place to prove to yourself that you can overcome your own limitations and transcend boundaries you thought you had. That is the zone where you want to be.

Cardio in Weight Loss and Fitness

What is "Cardio" training? Cardio is short for "cardiovascular" training. There are many ways to categorize cardio training. Although cardio training is also typically used interchangeably with the term "aerobic" training, they are technically not the same thing. Aerobic training is "training which elicits aerobic metabolism at a higher ratio than anaerobic metabolism." [73] Cardio training is training that conditions the cardiovascular system. Cardiovascular training can be either aerobic or anaerobic. At higher intensities, cardio training becomes more and more anaerobic. Cardio training at lower intensities is more aerobic.

In more simple terms, "aerobic" training refers to training that uses oxygen as the catalyst for the metabolic pathways fueling the energy required to complete the training. It is generally lower intensity activity than the all-out, super-intense activity of much of the fitness zeitgeist these days featuring terms like "crushed it" or "killing it". There are several levels or zones of cardio training. In general terms, many health and fitness experts explain that cardio training begins at a level above 50% of your maximum heart rate (MHR).

An easy way to calculate your MHR is to subtract your age from 220. There is a more individualized and complicated way to obtain a specific number for yourself, but for our purposes, the age method works well enough. Using that equation, a 45-year old man has a MHR of 175.

Above 80% of MHR, you transition into the anaerobic zone. Therefore, above 50% MHR and below 80% MHR is the range that defines what is known as the "aerobic zone" (AZ). We will refer to it from this point on as the AZ. Though not every health or fitness expert agrees on this exact range for the AZ, there is a general consensus around these numbers. Why you should care about AZ, is that it is the zone where fat is used as the primary fuel driving the activity you are engaged in. To get ripped, you must get rid of fat.

Within the AZ is a specific heart rate at which Maximal fat oxidation (MFO) occurs. This varies widely by individual, but in a 2009 study by the Health and Human Performance Laboratory at the University of St. Thomas and published in *The Journal of Strength and Conditioning Research*, evaluating 36 fit runners (20 male), MFO occurred in all the individuals between 60% and 80% of MHR. [74] To discover your exact MFO heart rate, you would have to have a laboratory evaluation performed.

The study made a point of evaluating the difference between the AZ and the fat burning zone (FBZ). For the fit runners in the study, the AZ occurred between 67.6% MHR and 87.1% MHR while the upper limit of the FBZ, as indicated above was 80% MHR. [75]

But wait a second, I thought the AZ and FBZ were basically the same thing? Not exactly. To understand the distinction, we must understand some basics about the metabolic energy systems that are responsible for delivering energy to our body's cells during different kinds of activity. Fundamentally, there are two basic energy delivery systems within our bodies as alluded to above: the aerobic (or oxygen-catalyzed) system and the anaerobic (or non-oxygen catalyzed system).

However, there are three different sources of energy that the body uses for fuel: fat, glucose, and adenosine triphosphate-phosphocreatine (ATP-PC). Both the aerobic system and the anaerobic system use two of the three different fuel sources available to the body. The aerobic system can use both fat and glucose. The anaerobic system can use glucose and ATP-PC.

The body will utilize different energy delivery systems (aerobic or anaerobic) and fuel sources depending primarily on how much energy is required and how quickly the body needs it. In a sense, this system acts as four distinct "gears" for the body in a similar way that a car or a bike has different gears depending on what the driver or rider is demanding of it. An important difference, though, is that all of the gears "are utilized concurrently, it is not like driving a car with a manual transmission, where you switch from one gear to another; *they are all used at all times.* However, as you change exercise intensities their relative contribution" to total energy supplied changes." [76]

The first gear of the system is the aerobic system burning fat metabolized by oxygen. This is also called aerobic "lipolysis". Since fat oxidation is a relatively slow process, it is used by the body during lower-intensity activities like walking or long-duration running. For example, in a fasted state (no food for the past 8-12 hours) during low-intensity exercise like walking at 2.5

to 3.0 miles per hour, "most of the energy need is provided by oxidation of" fat. [77]

As exercise intensity increases to approximately 65% VO$_2$max (which is just under 80% MHR)[78] or a moderate intensity level, fat burning peaks. However, fat cannot sustain all the demands of exercise at that intensity level, so the body begins shifting to its second gear: "aerobic glycolysis". This is where oxygen is utilized by the body to burn glucose (as opposed to fat). In this state, "about one-half of the total energy is simultaneously derived from" glucose. [79]

If you were to eat a meal containing carbohydrates prior to exercise (instead of being fasted), fat-burning is blunted but exercise performance is improved. [80] Why? Because, "the human body bases the order in which it burns the fats, carbohydrates and protein you give it on three factors: How many cells require it, how much effort it takes to convert it to usable energy and how much it can store. Your body burns carbohydrates before fat because they score well in all three categories." [81]

This is an important consideration when planning your workouts: is the goal of your workout on a given day to burn fat or to perform well in your workout? If the objective is fat-burning, performing the workout in a fasted state can possibly help burn more fat. However, like many issues in fitness, there is also evidence to the contrary: "there's at least one study showing that the amount of fat burned during the 24-hour recovery period is significantly greater when trainees ate a meal before the workout." [82] As a noteworthy aside, your body cannot burn carbohydrates directly. It must convert them to glucose first.

The anaerobic system, like the aerobic system, also has two different "gears". The first "gear" of the anaerobic system is called the ATP-PC system. "This energy system relies on ATP that is stored in the muscle, which is then released rapidly when needed. The system is highly dependent on creatine phosphate, which is why power and speed athletes often supplement with creatine. The system can recover quickly, usually within three to five minutes." [83] The ATP stored in the muscles that fuels the initial burst of energy from the ATP-PC system "last[s] only a few seconds after which the breakdown of PC provides energy for another 5-8 seconds of activity. Combined, the ATP-PC system can sustain all-out exercise for up to 10-15 seconds and it is during this time that the potential rate for power output is at its greatest" relative to all other sources of energy for the body. [84]

The second "gear" within the anaerobic system is called the "anaerobic glycolysis system". It is also sometimes called the "lactic acid system" because lactic acid is the by-product of anaerobic glycolysis. When you "feel the burn" while working out, you know that your body is using anaerobic glycolysis, and lactic acid is building up in your muscle tissue. The lactic acid causes the burning sensation. Anaerobic glycolysis occurs as exercise increases in intensity and the energy demands of the body exceed the ability of the body to deliver oxygen to catalyze the burning of glucose as an energy source.

> In those cases, the working muscles generate energy anaerobically. This energy comes from glucose through a process called glycolysis, in which glucose is broken down or metabolized into a substance called pyruvate through a series of steps. When the body has plenty of oxygen, pyruvate is shuttled to an aerobic pathway to be further broken down for more energy. But when oxygen is limited, the body temporarily converts pyruvate into a substance called lactate, which allows glucose breakdown—and thus energy production—to continue. The working muscle cells can continue this type of anaerobic energy production at high rates for one to three minutes, during which time lactate can accumulate to high levels. [85]

To summarize what we have learned so far about "cardio", the body can use three energy sources as fuel and four different

43

"gears" to deliver energy to the body. Who knew there was so much to it?

But we started the examination of the body's different "gears" when we began discussing the difference between the AZ and the FBZ. Now, we can approach the issue with more clarity. In the study we considered at the beginning of this section, the researchers discovered the maximum calories burned per minute in the FBZ was 11.5 *total* calories per minute, while the maximum *total* calories burned per minute in the AZ was 14.2. On the other hand, the researchers found that the number of *fat calories* burned at the peak of the FBZ was 3.45 calories per minute while the *fat calories* burned at the peak of the AZ was 1.68 calories per minute. [86] Realize that your calorie burn numbers may not match the numbers of the fit runners in this study. If you are in poor to moderate condition, you may only burn 50-60% of the calories that they burned. [87]

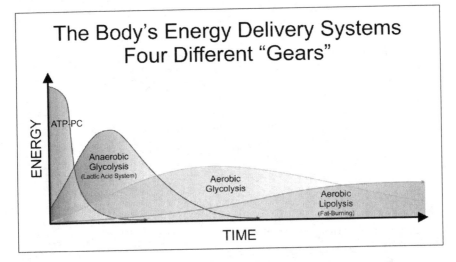

All of this is very interesting. Another study from 1993 found similar results: total fat oxidation rose steadily as exercise intensity increased from 25% VO_2max (approximately 53% MHR) to 65% of VO_2max (approximately 79% MHR), but then began declining as intensity increased further. At 85% VO_2max (approximately 91% MHR), fat burning was at the same level as 25% VO_2max. [88] All of this has implications for the way we train. About their findings, the researchers from the first study remarked:

> If the objective is metabolism of fat calories, training at the upper limits of AZ should not be recommended. If total caloric expenditure is the objective, the upper limits of AZ will be the most efficient. In addition to more calories being expended during exercise, caloric expenditure during recovery from high-intensity exercise is greater than recovery caloric expenditure from low-intensity exercise because of the additional energy requirement of ventilation, restoration of adenosine triphosphate phosphocreatine, replenishment of glycogen stores, and body temperature elevation. Also, prolonged exercise at high intensity, as in marathon running, has shown a gradual decrease in carbohydrate oxidation and gradual increase in fat oxidation as glycogen stores become depleted. If fat calories, and not total calories, were a better predictor of weight control, we would expect endurance athletes, who spend a rather large volume of training above FBZ, to have weight control problems. This is clearly not the case. [89]

Another important point to make about "cardio" training, is that it is possible to be in shape anaerobically but in poor aerobic condition. The gravity of our societal milieu today seems to pull us inexorably toward the idea that our workouts must be nasty, brutish, and ... intense ... every time. In terms of cardio workouts, that tends to lead many of us to fail to develop our aerobic conditioning since it is much less intense than anaerobic conditioning. To fully develop the long-term health and longevity benefits of physical fitness, we must be fit both aerobically and anaerobically. "Many people, especially many 'athletes' are running long distances with a very poor aerobic system, relying heavily on their anaerobic system to get them through their training. This anaerobic training is their 'cardio' and it's very,

very unhealthy, which is part of the reason so many point to 'cardio' as harmful to one's health, especially when it comes to the immune and hormonal systems." [90]

This is a trap I personally have fallen into: I often feel like I need to go hard every time in my workouts which pulls me out of the aerobic zone. I often cannot help myself from cranking up my own personal intensity level. It is an issue I am working on; too many "Just Do It" commercials seen in my youth. In all seriousness, though, I have disturbingly noticed that, while I can run 4.5 miles in about 30 minutes, I am often out of breath while talking on a relatively mild walk. That is evidence of a poorly conditioned aerobic system. Eventually, that will bite me if I do not begin to seriously address it.

In a 1990 study published in the *Journal of Psychosomatic Research*, groups of police officers were assigned to an aerobic conditioning, anaerobic conditioning, or control group. After ten weeks of training, the aerobic training group "evinced larger changes on the self-report measures of well-being and stress than the anaerobic trainers". [91] So, throughout this book, the case has clearly been made that anaerobic training (mostly in the form of resistance training) is critical. It is. But as unsexy as it might be, do not neglect your aerobic conditioning. That can mean just going out for a nice, briskly-paced walk on a regular basis.

Before we wrap up this section on cardio training, there are a few more important points to make. Always do your cardio training after your resistance training session. The reason for this is two-fold. First, cardio training prior to a resistance training session negatively impacts your ability to perform during resistance training. A 2016 study from *The Journal of Strength and Conditioning Research* stated, "acute resistance exercise performance is significantly compromised in healthy men after aerobic exercise of different type, intensity, and duration with largest reductions observed after high-intensity interval exercise." [92] The second reason is that after the first 30 minutes of your resistance training session, your body's "glycogen and blood glucose have been used up and the body uses primarily fatty acids for its fuel. Switching to moderate intensity exercise lets the body consume free fatty acids for metabolic energy and gives the body time to remove the lactic acid so that aerobic exercise can be performed." [93] This is a key to getting ripped. By performing cardio after resistance exercise, you are allowing your body to have maximum energy as it powers through the body's supplies of immediately available energy. Then, free fatty acids are down-regulated from the body's fat stores. During the remainder of your resistance session and during your cardio session, you will be burning off these free fatty acids from stored body fat as opposed to allowing your body to up-regulate them back into stored body fat.

Preeminent experts such as Dr. Jacob Wilson of the Applied Science and Performance Institute and Associate Editor of the Journal of Strength and Conditioning Research highly endorse cardio training: "if you want a shredded physique, cardio is a must ... if you want single digit body fat, you are going to have to incorporate cardio". Importantly, Dr. Wilson recommends avoiding performing cardio training on your lower body days: "training the lower body on the same day as cardio will hurt your gains. Therefore, separate cardio from legs by at least 24 to 48 hours." Performing steady-state cardio training on the same day as working legs can result in a loss of muscle mass rather than an overall gain. Finally, "cardio done for more than 20-30 minutes impairs muscle gains more, which means I would recommend keeping your cardio short and intense ... I would never go over 30 minutes of low-intensity cardio more than four days per week. Start low and progress upward. Also, do not forget to use HIIT ..." [94]

Which is the perfect segue way into our next topic...

High-Intensity Interval Training

The key to cardio is to consider HIIT training, which we will discuss next, and to limit it to about 15-20 minutes. Doing more than that is not only ineffective, but it is going to decrease the time you must spend building muscle via resistance exercise.

High-intensity interval training is not a new concept in fitness, but it is certainly one that needs to be part of any Dad's workout routine. As briefly mentioned above, this is a way to pack cardio workouts into relatively small-time slots, allowing you to get your heart rate into the fat burning zone, and to boost those periods of very high-intensity work, to get muscle fibers firing.

"HIIT is a great form of cardiovascular training because it skyrockets your metabolism (you burn more calories) and increases your oxygen demand after training (you burn more calories for a longer period of time). In addition to that, you are able to fit a large amount of work into a very small window of time." [95] Additionally, for men over the age of 45, the good news is that a 2017 study discovered that, "six weeks' HIIT improves peak power output in masters athletes and increases free testosterone." [96] "Masters" athletes are athletes over the age of 35.

Recommendations for the exercise to rest ratio during HIIT training vary. A 2014 study from the *Journal of Strength and Conditioning Research* determined a "2:1 work-to-rest ratio is optimal during HIIT". [97] In other words, the high-intensity interval will be twice as long as the short rest period. On the other hand, according to Master Strength and Conditioning Coach Tom Kelso, the ratio can vary all the way up to 1 to 3 for longer work periods. [98] That would mean, for example, 1.5 minutes of intense running followed by 4.5 minutes of rest. It is possible to use your own design in HIIT training and it can include treadmills, ellipticals, running, swimming or even doing basic types of exercises such as squats, burpees, or push-ups. It is even possible to combine exercise options during the workout phase.

One of the most widely known methods for performing a HIIT workout is called the Tabata Protocol. It is based on research conducted by Dr. Izumi Tabata, dean of the Graduate School of Sport and Health Science at Ritsumeikan University in Japan. In 1996, Dr. Tabata tested two groups of physically active young men over six weeks training on stationary bikes. The first group was subjected to steady-state endurance training five days per week for an hour each training session. The second group also trained five days per week. On four of those days, they performed HIIT with seven to eight 20-second cycles of maximum intensity exercise and 10 seconds of rest for a total exercise time of 3.5 minutes to 4 minutes. After six weeks, the results showed that the HIIT group had improved both their aerobic and anaerobic fitness more than the steady-state exercisers. [99] That was an unexpected result of the experiment. It showed that in four minutes of HIIT it was possible to beat the results of one hour of steady-state exercise. That is encouraging.

However, a 2015 study published in the *Journal of Sports Science and Medicine* confounds Tabata's results. "This study compared the effects of two HIIT protocols vs steady-state training on aerobic and anaerobic capacity following 8-weeks of training." [100] In this study, the sedentary participants were assigned to three groups exercising three times per week. One group exercised at a steady-state for 20 minutes, the next group did HIIT for 20 minutes using a cycle of 30 seconds of hard intensity (as opposed to maximum intensity in the Tabata protocol) and 60 seconds off. The last group performed the Tabata protocol. After eight weeks, aerobic and anaerobic fitness increased in all groups, but "the main finding of this study was the substantial equivalence of increases in measures of both aerobic and anaerobic exercise performance in all three training groups. Contrary to the frequent claims in the literature of larger responses following high-intensity exercise training regimes, in this group of relatively untrained young adults there was no

apparent advantage gained from more intense exercise".
Additionally, of the three protocols in this study, the participants
least enjoyed the Tabata protocol. [101]

A third study performed in 2006 found results similar to the 2015
study above. Sixteen active, young men were placed into two
groups for six sessions of training over two weeks: one
performing sprint-interval training (SIT) and the other group
performing volume endurance training (ET). The SIT group
performed four to six cycles of 30 seconds of maximum intensity
effort followed by four minutes of rest. The ET group cycled for
90-120 minutes. After the study, both groups had similar results.
The researchers concluded that: HIIT "is a time-efficient strategy
to induce rapid adaptations in skeletal muscle and exercise
performance that are comparable to" endurance training. [102]

So, research has found that HIIT using cycles anywhere from 20
seconds of maximum intensity effort followed by 10 seconds of
rest to 30 seconds of activity followed by four minutes of rest can
produce fitness improvements equivalent to or better than much
longer bouts of endurance training. What the HIITT training
regimens have in common is their maximum intensity effort.
"The goal is to practice the exercises with maximal intensity for a
short duration of time. Don't worry about your feelings of guilt
for not working out longer. Doing more than the specified four to
eight sets will not help you in the long run." [103]

One of the most important reasons to include HIIT in your
getting-ripped repertoire is the short period of time required to
complete it and still reap the benefits of endurance exercise that
requires up to 15 times longer to complete. That allows you to
devote more time to other important areas of your life.
Additionally, HIIT training boosts your metabolism in the 24
hours following a session to a similar degree as much longer
endurance exercise bouts. [104]

Do not perform HIIT every day. In fact, most trainers
recommend avoiding back to back days of HIIT Avoid doing HIIT-

focused exercises that are geared towards the same area of the body as your weight lifting program for the day.

Sample HIIT Schedule 1 (Tabata Protocol):
Four days/week sprint or cycle training
Four minutes total
20 seconds MAXIMUM intensity effort
10 seconds rest
Seven to eight cycles as able

Sample HIIT Schedule 2:
Four days/week sprint or cycle training
20 - 27 minutes total
30 seconds MAXIMUM intensity effort
Four minutes rest
Four to six cycles as able

What Is the Ideal Training Program?

One of the first things that everyone starting in the gym wants to see is a simple, easy and completely doable schedule for working out. They also want to get the maximum amount of results for the minimum amount of time, without any pain, hard work or having to give up a few of the things they may have come to enjoy.

The reality is, there is no way to become a ripped dad after 45 if you are not willing to put in the work and to sacrifice. That may not be what you want to hear, but it is the truth. As I have told my son many times as he has grown up, "Life demands a price. You either pay now or pay later. It is much more expensive to pay later because life charges interest". You need to understand that. My son, by the way, took that lesson to heart, applied himself, and is now at Harvard on a four-year scholarship. You can reap similar benefits physically if you heed that advice.

You can ignore working out and healthy eating today and tomorrow. No one will stop you from doing that. Eventually, though, it will catch up with you. The scientific research is irrefutable: exercise and a good diet cause you to live longer and healthier:

- "Change in physical fitness in healthy middle-aged men is a strong predictor of mortality. Even small improvements in physical fitness are associated with a significantly lowered risk of death." [105]
- "Total physical activity and mortality were inversely related in men. Vigorous but not nonvigorous activities were associated with longevity." [106]
- "The longer, harder and more often you exercise, the greater the health benefits, including reducing the risk of diseases such as cancer and diabetes, according to the recommendations [of the Department of Health and Human Services], which were based on a decade of scientific research." [107]
- "Recent and accumulating work in unicellular and invertebrate model organisms, rodents, monkeys, and humans indicates that diet has a much more pervasive and prominent role than previously thought in modulating mechanisms of aging and its associated diseases." [108]

There is no magic exercise routine or special supplement that will shed fat and build muscles: that must come from you working your body on a regular, routine schedule and sticking to a nutrition plan that nourishes your body with the right kinds of nutrients and with the right number of calories.

It also means starting where you are right now: good, bad, or ugly; as opposed to where you wish you were or where you think you should be. If you have not been intensively involved in working out for a while, you cannot immediately return to the same level you were at. Be smart. If you are fat and out of shape right now, it is fine. But be honest with yourself and start slowly. You will get better. But you must approach your situation intelligently. There is no point in going to the gym and lifting the heaviest possible weights or using terrible form because you do not know what you are doing yet and injuring yourself, resulting in days, weeks, or even months before you can start again. I have "been there and done that". It is not worth it.

Heed this advice: Professor Marcas Bamman Ph.D. of the University of Alabama in Birmingham cautions, "If you are a beginner, or haven't exercised for a while ... Don't try to immediately do what you could do 20 years ago at college or high school. He recommends cardiovascular exercises such as running and cycling three or four times a week and strength training twice a week." Professor Bamman emphasizes the importance of starting slowly and building your strength and fitness gradually to minimize the risk of injury. [109]

Different individuals have different lifestyles. Someone who works behind a desk all day, is moderately to significantly overweight, and is relatively inactive outside of work will need to start slower than someone who has a very active job, plays recreational sports, and has only a few pounds to lose.

Personally, after failing at several attempts at trying to get back in shape over the course of about one year due to trying to push myself too hard and ending up injured each time, I got smart: for several months I simply walked every day. I made it my goal to get 10,000 steps per day at first and worked up to 20,000 steps per day by the end of those several months. While walking I listened to hundreds of podcasts on diet, fitness, and health. All of that created the base of physical fitness and knowledge that allowed me to know how to eat right, get back in the gym in a sensible way, start doing some light weightlifting and some slow, short running. That, in turn, eventually turned into getting ripped.

The key to keep in mind is that getting started is the most important part. Get up and get yourself onto the walking trail, into the gym, or dojo, or "box", or wherever you are going to start down the path toward getting ripped. As author David Deida says in his book *The Way of the Superior Man*, "You are entirely responsible for cutting through your own laziness, addictions, and unclarity. There is nothing to wait for and nobody to blame ... it won't work, if, when it comes down to it, you'd rather masturbate, read the newspaper, or watch TV than cut through your addictions, discipline your daily life" and get yourself moving. [110]

Most gyms today will have a trainer as part of the service they offer. These individuals can help in setting up a reasonable training program that will start where you are currently and allow you to build toward a ripped body with a plan individually tailored to your specific situation. Strength and fitness coaches outside of gyms are available for hire. Some will consult with you online via email, phone, Skype, and/or text if they are not located close to you. I have personally used both a fitness and strength coach. They have helped me tremendously and short-cut my progression to my goals. In my opinion, coaches are invaluable.

It is a wise decision to also do your own research. Begin to become an expert. Learn how your body is responds to various kinds and amounts of activity, sleep, food, stress, light (circadian rhythms), etc. As your base of knowledge grows and you become more familiar with the nuances and needs of your body, make the necessary changes to customize your program to meet your needs.

One of the keys to making fitness work for you is to make it enjoyable and rewarding. For example, one way that I have come to love working out is by, as they say in the military, "embracing the suck". I am also able to enjoy visualizing myself maintaining my health and vigor well into old age as a result of my healthy lifestyle. Find aspects of working out and eating right that motivate you and fire you up. If you cannot find anything to appreciate about the process, it is much less likely you are going to stick with it.

The bottom line is that the ideal training program for you is going to be highly individualized to you. There are approximately three billion base pairs and 19,000 genes in the human genome. [111] Researchers are only at the dawn of beginning to comprehend the mind-bogglingly complex ways in which the human genome operates. Beyond that, innumerable environmental variables influence genetic expression in ways science is only beginning to understand. Each person is definitively unique. What works for one person may not work for another. While advice of a general nature can be offered, realize that ultimately, the ideal training program is going to be one that you discover for yourself as you grow in your fitness journey. Reading this book is a great start.

At the end of this chapter, you will find a section on monitoring and tracking your fitness. There are several very low-cost or even free options out there that can be very helpful in keeping you on-track and in control of your fitness, even if you are not going to work with a trainer and are making your quest to get ripped a do-it-yourself project.

What to Consider in Setting Up a Plan

When setting up a training plan, there are a few things to consider. One factor is what is known as periodization, or how to work through time in specific periods to maximize your muscle-building goals.

A traditional option is known as linear periodization. Linear periodization "divides a strength training program into different periods or cycles: macrocycles (9– 12 months), mesocycles (3–4 months), and microcycles (1– 4 weeks), gradually increasing the training intensity while decreasing the training volume within and between cycles". [112] In this training method, the volume (remember this is the total amount of weight lifted in a training session) will decrease over time while the intensity will increase (in weightlifting terms, intensity refers to the load – or amount – of weight). [113] In other words, at the beginning of a linear periodization training cycle, you will start with lighter loads and higher repetitions. As the cycle progresses, you will shift to heavier loads and lower repetitions. Think of this as working towards a competition where you train to build up both strength and stamina and then focus more specifically on strength as the competition nears. Here is an example of a linear periodization plan for a given exercise: Weeks 1-4; 3 sets of 12 repetitions, Weeks 5-8; 3 sets of 10 repetitions; Weeks 9-12; 4 sets of 8 repetitions. [114]

A 2009 study evaluated the effect of an eight-week, split-body (incorporating separate upper-body and lower-body workouts) linear periodization training program on college-aged and middle-aged men. The results should be particularly interesting to us middle-aged men: both bench press and leg press strength were "significantly increased" and lean body mass as measured by DEXA body composition scan (currently considered the gold standard in assessing body composition). Most interestingly, "middle-aged men lost significantly more fat mass and significantly decreased percent body fat compared with college-aged men". [115] By the way, that is the same study we referred to in the beginning of the book that showed middle-aged men could, in fact, pack on muscle – it turns out, using linear periodization.

Another option is non-linear periodization. In contrast to linear periodization, non-linear periodization "involves a dramatic variation of training volume and intensity in shorter periods of time, occurring frequently from one training session to the next" [116] Non-linear periodization is also referred to as "undulating periodization". A 2002 study by Arizona State University scientists evaluating the effectiveness of a linear periodization program versus a daily undulating periodization program concluded, "Making program alterations on a daily basis was

56

more effective in eliciting strength gains than doing so every 4 weeks". [117] A newer study in 2012 compared the results of a 12-week non-linear periodization program versus a linear periodization program. After compiling the results of the study, the scientists concluded, "our study suggests that, at least in trained subjects over a 12-week training period, the implementation of an [non-linear periodization] program may result in superior maximal strength and [muscle thickness] improvements compared with the classical [linear periodization] model. Additionally, the [non-linear periodization] model variations in volume and intensity occurring from one training session to the next may reduce the ''monotony' of performing repetitive training sessions and result in greater practitioner adherence." [118]

To give you an idea of what a daily non-linear periodization program looks like, here is a sample workout scheme:

- **Monday**: Deadlift, 5 sets of 3 repetitions at 70% 1RM; Bench Press, 4 sets of 4 repetitions at 85% 1RM; Squat, 3 sets of 10 at 70% 1RM
- **Wednesday**: Bench Press, 5 sets of 3 repetitions at 70% of 1 RM; Squat, 4 sets of 4 repetitions at 85% 1RM; Deadlift, 3 sets of 10 repetitions at 65% 1RM
- **Friday**: Squat, 5 sets of 3 repetitions at 70% 1RM; Deadlift, 4 sets of 4 repetitions at 85% 1RM; Bench Press, 3 sets of 10 repetitions at 70% 1RM
- **Saturday**: Pullups, 4 sets of 4-6 repetitions; Shoulder Press, 4 sets of 4-6 repetitions; Romanian Deadlift, 4 sets of 8 repetitions; Pushups, 3 sets of 15 repetitions; Goblet Squats, 3 sets of 12 repetitions [119]

While nonlinear periodization strategies are most commonly used by competitive athletes and more advanced weightlifters, they can be incorporated into your training as well. Keep things moving and changing. Look for new exercises to work into your routine and plan them strategically so they do not negate or minimize the gains you can achieve. Always strive to keep learning so that you can continuously improve your workout strategies.

Wait, What About CrossFit?

One of the latest in exercise trends over the last few years has been CrossFit. You have probably heard of this high-intensity fitness program. It has become a wildly popular fitness craze. As of 2016, according to business news outlet CNBC, "CrossFit has 13,000 gyms in more than 120 countries. That's more than the 12,521 Starbucks locations in the United States. Its direct rival, Planet Fitness, has just 1,124 locations." [120]

It was originally developed by Greg Glassman, an entrepreneur and former gymnast. CrossFit "is a training program that builds strength and conditioning through extremely varied and challenging workouts". [121] The intent of CrossFit is to build functional, broad-spectrum fitness as opposed to the specialized, possibly out-of-balance fitness CrossFit devotees would argue are produced by other workout programs. CrossFit gyms are called "boxes". CrossFit boxes typically cater to working adults. Over half of CrossFit participants earn incomes greater than $150,000 per year and 40% have graduate degrees. [122] Boxes usually have classes throughout the day as well as in the evenings, and they are usually open on the weekends for several classes.

One of the basic features of CrossFit is that each day there is a different "Workout of the Day", or in CrossFit parlance, "WOD". WOD's are a combination of different exercises. Typical exercises that comprise a WOD are power cleans, burpees, jumping pull-ups, deadlifts, box jumps, and kettlebell swings. Each day, a box will "prescribe" (or "Rx") a specific WOD for everyone attending the box that day. That means everyone at the box that day does the same WOD. CrossFit WOD's are designed from the bottom up for "scalability" which allows everyone from beginners to elite athletes to be challenged by the same WOD. The difference is that beginners and less advanced athletes do lighter weights or fewer sets and repetitions. [123] Or, if they are unable to complete the movement required by an exercise due to injury or disability, a similar movement can be substituted.

The fact that everyone at a WOD does their workout together is another key feature of CrossFit. It is a group exercise – with a competitive edge: according to the official CrossFit website: "Harnessing the natural camaraderie, competition and fun of sport or game yields an intensity that cannot be matched by other means. The CrossFit program is driven by data. Using whiteboards as scoreboards, keeping accurate scores and records, running a clock, and precisely defining the rules and standards for performance, we not only motivate unprecedented output but derive both relative and absolute metrics at every workout. This data has important value well beyond motivation." [124]

As explained, everything is counted and measured creating an atmosphere where peer pressure is generated to improve on personal bests. It also creates internal competition to keep up with or beat other CrossFitters performances, which helps to motivate many people.

Studies on CrossFit have shown that it is effective at improving fitness. A 2013 study conducted by researchers from Ohio State University concluded, "we can infer from our data that a crossfit-based HIPT [high-intensity power training] program can yield meaningful improvements of maximal aerobic capacity and body composition in men and women of all levels of fitness".

A 2010 study led by US Army researchers found, "after only six-weeks of training using the CrossFit program, on average the athletes increased their level of physical fitness by 20%. One athlete increased her level of fitness by 41%. Moreover, the athletes in this study experienced relatively equal increases across all of the four assessments each of which required a different type of conditioning and skill set." [125]

In 2015, Polish scientists determined that CrossFit improves VO_2max, body composition (less fat, more muscle), and increases levels of brain-derived neurotrophic factor, a protein vital to a healthy brain. [126]

Clearly, CrossFit can be beneficial. However, CrossFit has drawbacks. It is not the ideal choice for everyone. It does not allow you to specialize since you go to the box to do the prescribed exercise and nothing else. Additionally, since CrossFit is performed in a group, if you are more of an individual, you may feel like a duck out of water at a CrossFit box. Furthermore, if your schedule makes it difficult to get to your box's classes at their scheduled times, you may not be able to participate as much as you (or the group) would like you to.

CrossFit has also become a polarizing topic. It seems that people either love it or they hate it.

Regarding the pitfalls of CrossFit, Chris Heria, co-founder of calisthenics fitness program TheNX expounded, "The problem [with CrossFit] is that over the years, it has become to do as many reps as you can in as short amount of time as possible. Which would mean that the faster you do your reps in the shortest amount of time possible equals the more efficiency ... Now, the truth is anybody that has been training seriously for quite some time knows that doing an exercise as fast as you can in the shortest amount of time possible does not mean that you're going to become more efficient ... What actually gets you better, stronger, and more efficient is progressional training with proper form and proper technique ... I've had students come into my gym from a CrossFit gym being able to do 30 Kipping pull-ups in a row, sometimes 40, but yet they can't do simple, basic pull-ups." [127]

In an interview with TigerFitness.com about the down side of CrossFit, Marc Lobliner, Owner/CEO of MTS Nutrition and a professional strength and conditioning coach explained, "You're teaching people complex movements in a group setting ... Imagine trying to teach a group of 40-something housewives

60

how to do a proper snatch ... how to do a proper power clean ... deadlifts, even squats, any compound movement is something that when you're doing a rep, you need to focus on that rep because there's too many things in your chain that could get injured. Once your form breaks down on a squat, you're asking for trouble. Once your form breaks down on a deadlift, you're asking for trouble. And those are not even as close to complex as a snatch or a clean. So, I mean, you're taking a complex movement built into a complex movement and asking people to do it for weight, time, and velocity. You're just asking for injuries"

Mr. Lobliner continued to explain that the training required to become certified as a CrossFit trainer is minimal: "It's a Saturday course. Not even a full Saturday." He pointed out that professional trainers spend four years at college and often obtain advanced degrees in order to teach the types of complex movements involved with CrossFit. He proceded, "That's the problem with CrossFit. The problem is to make it mainstream, to make the cost of entry lower, to make it where it can expand fast they had to dumb down the certification. By dumbing down the certification, you increase the chance of injury. And that's what's happened." [128]

In an interview with CrossFit CEO Glassman, CBS News *60 Minutes* correspondent Sharyn Alfonsi asked him about the low barrier to entry for CrossFit box owners:

> One reason CrossFit's grown so fast is because just about anyone who wants to open a "box" can after paying a $3,000 yearly fee and passing a two-day seminar. It's how the company makes most of its money.
>
> Sharyn Alfonsi: "Two days to take a course, then I can open a gym?"
>
> Greg Glassman: Amazing, huh? [129]

However, a 2013 study determined, "Injury rates with CrossFit training are similar to that reported in the literature for sports such as Olympic weight-lifting, power-lifting and gymnastics and lower than competitive contact sports such as rugby union and rugby league. Shoulder and spine injuries predominate ..." [130]

On the other hand, the nature of the CrossFit organization's business structure makes it very difficult to obtain real data on injury rates within the world of CrossFit: "CrossFit, as a body, has no data collection mechanism. Think about this, because this becomes the loophole for anyone wishing to defend CrossFit's safety record. **The records don't exist ...** Because CrossFit is an affiliate system and not a franchisor, the system is less like the head-and-appendages body of a franchise and more like a solar system where the planets orbit loosely around the sun, albeit unattached. **Which means there is not now, nor can there ever practically be, any mechanism for reporting of injury data.** In a system where CrossFit HQ prides itself on little oversight of its affiliates - you buy the license to use their name and that is it - there is no possible way for CrossFit, Inc., to monitor injury rates or collect data." [131]

Something to be aware of is that in the 2017 regional CrossFit competitions leading up to the international CrossFit Games, 36 competitors withdrew from contention due to tears of their pectoral muscles during the regionals. [132]

There are additional issues with CrossFit that should be considered before deciding if this is the right type of training for you. First, many people find the training groups very intensive and challenging, particularly for someone new to the program. Remember, the goal is to do as much of something in the time period as possible, which as discussed above can set the conditions for incurring an injury if you are not using proper form especially as you become fatigued. If you are more focused on going fast than doing it right, there is a much greater risk for injury.

Additionally, the dynamic of performing in a group setting can lead to ego usurping wisdom. This too can lead to injuries as people go beyond where their quivering muscles are telling them is safe.

Think of this type of training as HIIT, but with a level of competition that makes it even more intense. CrossFit has been proven to be able to deliver an effective workout. Realize, though, that as a man in his mid-40's or older, injury avoidance has to be a primary concern. One study found that CrossFit participants reported an injury rate of 73.5% during CrossFit training. [133] An injury can set you back weeks, months, or even forever.

The *Ripped Dad* 12-Week Workout Program

Phase One Workouts

During Phase One of the **Ripped Dad** program you will be exercising 6 days per week. <u>As always, consult with a doctor before beginning any exercise program to ensure that you are ready to dive into intense activity</u>. Three of those workouts will involve a combination of compound resistance training and metabolic training. You will begin each of these workouts by doing 3 sets of 12 repetitions on a compound, multi joint resistance exercise. Your goal is to take approximately 40-50 seconds to complete the set. Your rest time between each set will be exactly 60 seconds.

If you are an absolute beginner to resistance training, your prime focus here is to train yourself in the proper form on these compound movements. Remember the focus is not only lifting a weight for a prescribed number of reps but on placing and sustaining tension on the working muscle. Start with just the bar and then progress within your own comfort zone until you are using 40-60% of your one rep max.

If you've been training with weight for a year or so, use 60-65% of your one rep max. You want to feel as if you still have a couple of reps left in you when you reach your 12 rep goal. Experienced trainers should go to 80% of their one rep max.

Once you have completed your 3 sets on this first exercise, you will then move to the metabolic part of the workout. You will be performing 4 exercises in succession. Each exercise will be done over the period of one minute and you will have a set number of reps to achieve within that minute. Any time left over within the minute is your rest time. For instance, if you have to do 25 prisoner squats and it takes you 43 seconds, then you have 17 seconds to recover before going to the next exercise.

You complete 8 consecutive rounds of the metabolic portion of the workout. That means that this portion will take up 32 minutes (4 x 1-minute workouts repeated 8 times). The initial compound exercise will take about 6 minutes (3 x 40-50 second sets with a 1-minute rest between sets).

In order to maximize your fat-burn, it is imperative that you stick to these times. To make this happen, you should have your workout equipment set out in your training space so you can move directly from one exercise to the next. You will obviously also need to have a timer clearly visible at all times.

If you are a beginner, your 8 rounds will follow this rep pattern .
. .

12 reps on each body weight exercise – 8 reps on each dumbbell exercise

If you have been working out for more than a year, your 8 rounds will follow this rep pattern . . .

15/15/15/12/12/12/10/10 reps on all bodyweight exercises – 8 reps on each dumbbell exercise

If you have been training for 2-3 years, your 8 rounds will follow this rep pattern . . .

20/20/20/15/15/15/12/12 reps on all bodyweight exercises – 8 reps on each dumbbell exercise

If you are an elite trainer, your 8 rounds will follow this rep pattern . . .

25/25/25/20/20/20/15/15 reps on all bodyweight exercises – 8 reps on each dumbbell exercise

The above designations are not locked in. Feel free to choose the rep count that provides you with the challenge level you need to get the workout that will bring the results you deserve. Over the course of the four weeks, you should be striving to move from one level to the next.

Workout Schedule

Week	Mon	Tues	Wed	Thurs	Fri	Sat	Sun
One	1a	HIIT	1b	HIIT	1c	HIIT	Rest
Two	1a	HIIT	1b	HIIT	1c	HIIT	Rest
Three	1a	HIIT	1b	HIIT	1c	HIIT	Rest
Four	1a	HIIT	1b	HIIT	1c	HIIT	Rest

Workout 1a

Compound Exercise

Squats 3 x 12

Metabolic Workout

Prisoner Squat

Bench Over
Jumping Jacks
Plank Rows

Workout 1b

Compound Exercise

Deadlift 3 x 12

Metabolic Workout

Cross Overs
Dumbbell Push Press
Power Jumps
Push Ups

Workout 1c

Compound Exercise

Dumbbell Bench Press 3 x 12

Metabolic Workout

Rocket Jumps
Plank Rows
Power Jumps

Phase One Progression Goal: To move up one rep count level over the four-week period. If you are already at the elite level, focus on adding 10% resistance to your dumbbell exercises over the 4 weeks.

Phase One HIIT Cardio

You will do HIIT cardio three times each week on alternate days. If you have access to a treadmill, exercise bike or rowing machine, you may use them. However, we will focus on using nothing but your own body for these sessions.

The basis of our HIIT sessions will be what is known as the Tabata Protocol as discussed earlier in *Ripped Dad: Fit After 45*. Recall that it involves 20 seconds of intense activity followed by a 10 second recovery period for multiple rounds.

Your HIIT sessions will be done on an open field or in a large room. They will involve sprinting at max speed for 20 seconds followed by a 10 seconds rest. Note that it is vital that you stick strictly to these times, which means that you will either be running with a stopwatch in hand or have someone on the sideline calling out 'Stop' and 'Start' to you.

Here is how your HIIT sprint sessions will proceed . . .

- Jog up and down for two minutes, alternating between high knees and butt kicks.
- When you get to 1:30 of your warm-up, start to mentally prepare for your first all-out sprint. Start moving your arms in more of a pumping action and pick up your pace.
- At precisely two minutes go directly into a full-on sprint. Imagine that you are being chased by a very large, very

hungry dog! Keep going at that pace for the entire 20 seconds.

- As soon as you hit 2:20 reduce to a walk (hands on hips!). Do this for exactly 10 seconds.
- At precisely 2:30, begin your second sprint. Your goal here is NOT to reduce the intensity of your last sprint.
- Repeat for the following number of rounds . . .
  - ➢ Beginner – 5 rounds
  - ➢ Intermediate – 7 rounds
  - ➢ Advanced – 8 rounds
  - ➢ Elite – 10 rounds

Over the course of the month, your progression goal is to add a round every week (so, if you are a beginner, you will be doing 5 rounds in week one, 6 rounds in week two, seven rounds in week three and 8 rounds in week four).

Phase Two Workouts

Workout Schedule

Week	Mon	Tues	Wed	Thurs	Fri	Sat	Sun
One	Upper Body A + Steady State	HIIT	Lower Body A + Steady State	HIIT	Upper Body B + Steady State	HIIT	Rest
Two	Lower Body B + Steady State	HIIT	Upper Body A + Steady State	HIIT	Lower Body A + Steady State	HIIT	Rest
Three	Upper Body B + Steady State	HIIT	Lower Body B + Steady State	HIIT	Upper Body A + Steady State	HIIT	Rest
Four	Lower Body A + Steady State	HIIT	Lower Body B + Steady State	HIIT	Upper Body B + Steady State	HIIT	Rest

Your Phase Two Workouts will take you through the second four weeks of the **Ripped Dad** program. You will be performing the same core exercises that you were introduced to in your Phase One workouts along with some additional moves.

During this 4-week phase, you will be alternating between different workouts. There are two upper body and two lower body workouts. The constant change up of moves will keep your mind in the game while also preventing your body from growing accustomed to the stresses being placed upon it.

Keep in mind that you will be working out with weights 3 times per week, not four. The program uses a two-day split routine. The body is divided into an upper body day and a lower body day. You train the abs every 2nd workout. Here are the four workouts that you will perform.

Upper Body Workout A

Exercise	Sets / Reps
Decline Dumbbell Row	3 x 10
Pull Ups	3 x 10
Barbell Bench Press	3 x 10
Dumbbell Incline Press	3 x 10
Dumbbell Lateral Raise	3 x 12
Dumbbell Shoulder Press	3 x 10
Lying Triceps Extension	3 x 10

Lower Body Workout A

Exercise	Sets / Reps
Squats	3 x 10
Farmer's Walk	3 x 12
Deadlift	3 x 10
Lying Leg Curl	3 x 10
Standing Calf Raise	3 x 12
Reverse Crunch	3 sets
Plank	3 x 15-20

Upper Body Workout B

Exercise	Sets / Reps
Decline Dumbbell Row	3 x 10, 1 set 20 (reduce weight)
Lat Pulldown	3 x 10
Side Lateral Raises	3 x 10
Incline Dumbbell Flies	3 x 10
Dumbbell Shoulder Press	3 x 12
Triceps Pushdown	3 x 10
Incline Dumbbell Curls	3 x 10

Lower Body Workout B

Exercise	Sets / Reps
Squats	3 x 10, 1 set 20 (reduce weight)
Leg Press	3 x 10, 1 set 20 (reduce weight)
Deadlift	3 x 10, 1 set 20 (reduce weight)
Lying Leg Curls	3 x 10
Standing Calf Raise	3 x 15
Kneeling Cable Crunch	3 x 15
Prone Superman	3 x 15

A Note on Resistance: Selecting the appropriate weight for each exercise will require a little bit of trial and error. For the first two weeks of the program your focus should be on training your body in correct exercise technique and performance. The resistance, therefore, can be a little lighter than optimum until you are in the groove of the movement.

Phase Two Cardio

During Phase Two you will be taking your cardio indoors 3X per week. You will be doing steady sate cardio for 20 minutes after each of your 3 weekly weight training workouts. You can use a treadmill, stair-climber, cycle or any other type of cardio equipment in the gym. Keep within the fat burning zone for the entire 20 minutes.

On your non-gym days, you will continue with your HIIT training. This time, however, you will do it in the form of a 25-minute run. You will jog for four minutes and then sprint for 30 seconds. At the end of this max effort sprint, walk to recover for one minute, then break back to a light jog for two minutes. Then immediately go back to a 30-second sprint. Your goal is to continue this pattern until your 25 minutes is up.

Phase Three Workouts

Workout Schedule

Week	Mon	Tues	Wed	Thurs	Fri	Sat	Sun
One	Chest / Triceps	HIIT 1	Back / Biceps	HIIT 2	Legs / Shoulders	HIIT 1	Rest
Two	Chest / Triceps	HIIT 2	Back / Biceps	HIIT 1	Legs / Shoulders	HIIT 2	Rest
Three	Chest / Triceps	HIIT 1	Back / Biceps	HIIT 2	Legs / Shoulders	HIIT 1	Rest
Four	Chest / Triceps	HIIT 2	Back / Biceps	HIIT 1	Legs / Shoulders	HIIT 2	Rest

During the final Phase of the **Ripped Dad** program, you will be performing a split routine resistance program. This will involve working one major body-part (chest, back, legs), paired with one minor body-part (biceps, triceps, shoulders) per workout. During this final phase, you will be lifting heavier, with a rep range between 6-8. This is your optimum muscle building and strength zone and you want to push to the limit on these workouts. Your days of keeping a couple of reps in the tank are over. Push to the limit – but never sacrifice good form. You should still be taking 40-50 seconds for every set in order to maximize time under tension.

You will be doing 3 resistance workouts per week on Monday, Wednesday and Friday as follows. . .

Monday – Chest / Triceps

Wednesday – Back / Biceps

Friday – Legs / Shoulders

72

Here are your workouts . . .

Chest / Triceps

Exercise	Sets / Reps
Dumbbell Bench Press	3 x 6-8
Incline Press	3 x 6-8
Incline Flies	3 x 12
Push Ups	2 x as many as possible
Triceps Pushdowns	3 x 8-10
Close Grip Bench Press	3 x 6-8

Back / Biceps

Exercise	Sets / Reps
Deadlift	3 x 6-8
Decline Dumbbell Row	3 x 6-8
Pull Ups	3 x as many as possible
Face Pulls	2 x 12
Barbell Curl	3 x 6-8
Incline Dumbbell Curls	3 x 8-10

Legs / Shoulders

Exercise	Sets / Reps
Squats	3 x 6-8
Farmer's Walk	3 x 10

Lying Leg Curls	3 x 8-10
Shoulder Press	3 x 6-8
Standing Calf Raises	3 x 15

Phase Three Cardio

Your Phase Three Cardio will follow a similar pattern as in Phase Two, with 20 minutes of steady state cardio following every resistance workout. On three non-gym days, you will perform HIIT training. You will alternate between the Tabata 20-second on, 10 seconds off training you did in Phase One (HIIT1) with the 25-minute sprint / jog / walk training from Phase Two (HIIT2). Keep pushing to work as hard as you can during each session.

Optimized Exercise Descriptions

Phase One Exercises

Bench-overs

Stand in the middle and to the side of a flat bench. Grab the sides of the bench as you bend your knees slightly. Now hop both feet up and over the bench to land softly on the other side. Your upper body should stay centered over the bench at all times. You want to achieve a soft, springy landing.

Cross-overs

Straddle a line on the floor (you can place a rolled-up towel down) with your feet close to each other. The right foot should be crossed in front of the left on the left side of the line and the left foot behind the right one on the right side of the line. Begin by jumping and simultaneously crossing your feet, landing with your right foot on the right side of the line and the left foot on the left side of the line. Immediately jump again, this time with the left foot crossed in front of the right foot on the right side of the line and vice versa. Make it your goal to land softly as you go through your reps.

Rocket Jumps

Stand with your hands positioned at chest level. Drop down into a squat position so that your thighs are parallel to the floor. Now, explosively reverse your position and move into a jump. As your feet clear the ground, move your hands together over your heads and reach up. Land softly on the balls of your feet.

Dumbbell Push Press

Stand with a pair of dumbbells at shoulder level, palms facing forward. Load for the press by dropping your hips and lowering to a quarter squat. Now explosively power the dumbbells overhead. Lock out at the top and keep your core tight throughout.

Jumping Jacks

Stand with your feet together and arms by your side. Now simultaneously jump your legs as far apart as possible and bring your hands overhead to clap above you. Quickly return to the start position.

Prisoner Squats

Start in a standing position with your fingers interlaced behind your head (prisoner position). Squat down, ensuring that your knees do not go over your toes. In the bottom you want your thighs to be parallel to the ground and the chest in an upright position. Now push through your legs to return to the start position.

Push Ups

Get down into a plank position with your hands flat on the ground beneath your shoulders and your legs straight, balancing on your toes. Start by engaging your core and lowering down to the floor until your elbows are bent at approximately 90 degrees. From here, power back up to the start of the plank, exploding from the chest. Be sure that your back does not sag throughout the movement.

Plank Rows

Drop down into a push up position with dumbbells in your hands. Begin in the top push up position with your arms fully extended and your body in a prone position. Now row one arm up to your side. Alternate rows from side to side. Both sides equal one rep.

Power Jumps

Stand with feet shoulder width apart and arms by your sides. Load your body by dropping into a quarter squat and explode into the air driving your knees up high. Immediately you come down, go directly into the next jump.

Lunge Press Ups

Start in a standing position with a pair of dumbbells resting on your shoulders. Lunge forward with the dumbbells on your shoulders. At the bottom of the lunge position, press the dumbbells overhead to full extension. Bring the dumbbells back down to the shoulders before pushing back up into the starting position. Repeat on the other leg.

Phase Two Exercises

UPPER BODY: Workout A

Exercise 1: **Decline Dumbbell Row**

Prime Mover: Latissimus dorsi, center and lower trapezius

76

This exercise is a modification of the standard bent over barbell row. It allows you to optimally work the large muscles of your back while minimizing the stress on your lower spine that is an inherent part of the barbell version of the exercise.

Begin by adjusting an incline bench to a low angle, about 20 or 30 degrees. If your gym doesn't have an adjustable bench, use a regular flat bench and put the rear legs up on a block. Make sure the bench is stable before beginning the exercise.

Lean over the high end of the bench so you're supporting yourself on your abdominals. To start with, the dumbbells should be slightly in front of you at about a 45-degree angle (like airplane wings). Grip them, palms facing back. Bend your elbows enough so that your shoulder blades travel out as far as they will go. The idea here is to ensure maximum range of motion for your lats and your middle / lower traps.

When you're in the correct position, you will feel a stretch across your middle back as well as in your lats.

Pull the weights up and back with the lift coming from your lats and traps, not your arms or shoulders. Concentrate on starting the movement by bringing your shoulder blades together and away from your head. As you pull, raise your chest slightly off the bench, but keep your abdominals firmly pressed against the bench to keep the pressure off your lower back. Rotate your wrists so that your palms end up facing one another. Keep your elbows close to your sides. Lift until your elbows are at waist level.

It's important that you mentally pull back and not just up. The combination of starting with the weights in front of you and pulling back activates the lower lats and ensures development of this difficult to reach area.

If you feel like you are doing a curl, you are doing this exercise incorrectly. Except for your grip, your forearms and biceps should be as relaxed as possible. Feel for the tension in your lower lats and center back. That's the key.

Next step: Reverse the motion to lower the weights. The dumbbells should end up not quite as far forward as they started, and not touching the ground. As you lower the weight, rotate your wrists so the dumbbells return to their initial 45-degree angles to the edge of the bench. Keep your elbows bent so you get the maximum stretch across the center back and in the lower abs. Remember to lean against the bench throughout the exercise to keep the strain off your lower back.

Exercise 2: **Pull Ups**

Prime Mover: Latissimus dorsi

Grab a chinning bar with an underhand, shoulder width grip, and hang with your elbows slightly bent. Pull your chin up above the bar, hold for a second or two, and lower your body with control. Let your legs hang straight down and don't jerk your way up. Just pull yourself up in a smooth motion and then let your body down under control.

For maximum stretch and contraction, lower yourself to the very bottom of each rep and pull up until your chin touches or goes above the bar.

If you are unable to perform one complete repetition on a chinning bar, start by doing reverse pushups. Perform reverse pushups as follows:

Fix a bar 1 meter above the ground (you can do this on a Smith machine). Lie down so that the bar is directly over your chest. Grab the bar with an overhand grip that's slightly wider than shoulder width. Lift your torso and legs off the floor so that only the back of your heels remains planted on the floor. Pull in your abs and hold your body in a straight line from head to heels.

Exercise 3: **Barbell Bench Press**

Prime Mover: Pectorals

Load the appropriate weight onto the bar. Lie on the bench and take a grip just wide enough so your forearms are not quite parallel. Too narrow a grip shifts the load onto the triceps and makes it difficult to feel the tension in the chest. Now pinch your shoulder blades together. Lower the bar to sternum level. Your elbows should end up at a 70-degree angle to your sides and your forearms should be vertical. Touch your chest (never bounce), forcefully

stretch your pecs and immediately drive upwards, squeezing your lats and arcing the bar up to its start position at mid-chest. Lock out briefly between reps. Keep your shoulders down throughout the movement.

Breathing: Inhale while the bar is overhead, hold your breath during the descent and breathe as your press back.

Exercise 4: **Dumbbell Incline Press**

Prime Mover: Pectorals

If the incline bench you are using is adjustable, set it to a 30-degree angle. Sit on the bench with a dumbbell in each hand. Rest the dumbbells on your thighs close to your knees. Kick up your legs, one at a time, to assist getting the weights into position up at your shoulders.

Press the dumbbells up, using your pecs to pull them up and across your chest. Keep your back flat against the bench as you lift. At the top of the movement, squeeze the pecs tightly and hunch your shoulders forward. Don't touch the weight together at the top of the exercise - keep them 2-3 inches apart. Slowly lower the weight down as far as you can, getting the greatest stretch possible.

Exercise 5: **Dumbbell Lateral Raise**

Prime Mover: Deltoids

Grasp a light pair of dumbbells with a closed, neutral grip. Stand with feet shoulder width apart. Hold the dumbbells out from the sides of your thighs with your palms facing inwards. Slightly flex your elbows and hold them in that position throughout the movement.

Now lift the dumbbells up and out to the sides with your hands, forearms, elbows and upper arms rising together. Do not shrug your shoulders to lift the weights. Keeping your body erect with your knees slightly flexed and feet flat on the floor, bring the dumbbells back to the starting position.

Exercise 6:

Dumbbell Shoulder Press

Prime Mover: Deltoids

Sit on a bench and grasp a pair of dumbbells with a closed, pronated grip. Your head should be up and your upper back and hips should be pressed against the back pad of the seat. Move the dumbbells to position them at

shoulder level with your palms facing forward. The dumbbell handles should be in line with each other and parallel to the floor.

Push the dumbbells up until your elbows are fully extended. Keep your wrists straight and directly above your elbows. Make sure, too, that you maintain your erect position. Do not lean back or lift off the bench as you press the dumbbells overhead.

Now lower the dumbbells back to the start position. Keep your wrists straight and directly above your elbows.

Exercise 7:

Lying Triceps Extension

Prime Mover: Triceps Lie on a flat bench with a barbell across your thighs. Position yourself so that the base of your head is against the end of the bench (in other words, so most of your head is off the bench). Grab the barbell with a narrow, palm down grip and kick your legs back to get the bar into position above your head.

Your arms should not be straight up and down. Rather, they should be inclined slightly backward and toward the head. This angle keeps tension on the triceps throughout the entire exercise. Bend your knees and hook your feet against the end of the bench.

Starting in this position, lower the bar to your forehead, keeping your forearms parallel to each other and your upper arms stationary. Don't allow the elbows to drift apart. Non-parallel forearms greatly decrease the effectiveness of the exercise and increase the strain on your elbows. Press the bar back up to the inclined position. Concentrate on keeping your upper arms parallel.

Exercise 8: **Standing Supinated Dumbbell Curls**

Prime Mover: Biceps Begin with a dumbbell in each hand, palms facing forward. You can increase your stability and decrease general strain during this exercise by performing this movement leaning against a bench with your knees slightly bent. Think of the exercise as a combination of two movements that must be smoothly integrated. The first is supination of the forearm. This involves rotating your forearm so that your palm, which begins facing backward, ends up facing forward.

Second is a curl. Proper curling is not obvious, nor is it what the body does naturally if given a chance. The natural tendency with any exercise is to do as little work as possible. When doing curls, for example, your body adjusts to the position of greatest mechanical advantage, taking as much strain off your biceps as possible - not at all what you want to get lean, fat free upper arms.

To maximize the work done by the biceps during any curl you need to: (1) Make sure that your elbow and arm remain in the ideal plane throughout the movement (perpendicular to your body). You don't want your elbows to move away from the body. (2) Keep your elbow slightly in front of you during the curl. The natural tendency is to let the elbow move next to the body - or worse yet, behind the body - as you raise the weight. This takes the strain off the biceps.

When performing a supinated curl, both the supination of the forearm and the curling motion should occur simultaneously. The supination should not happen all at once. Try to rotate the forearm smoothly throughout the entire curling motion. A common error is to do the entire supination at the beginning of the movement.

Remember to bring your elbow slightly forward as you do the curl - not back, or to the side. Keeping your elbow in front of you ensures maximum action of the long head of the bicep, which flexes the shoulder as well as the elbow. Lean into the curl t the top of the movement to keep the tension on the biceps.

On the way down, it's important to exactly reverse the movement performed on the way up. Don't let your elbows drift from their position slightly in front of you. Much of the benefit of any exercise come from returning to the start position. You throw the benefit away if your form is sloppy when lowering the weight.

LOWER BODY:

Workout A

Exercise 1: **Squats**

Prime Mover: Quadriceps

Use extreme caution with the squat. This is a compound movement. It's always important to nail the form on a movement, but it is doubly important with squats. Avoid injury! Use no weight or light weights until you have the movement mastered!

Stand in front of a squat rack with an Olympic bar loaded to the desired weight and set at the level of your shoulders. Position yourself under the bar so that it is resting across your traps. Take one step back still staying within the rack. Your feet should be a little wider than shoulder width and your toes pointing outward.

Keep your back straight, your chest thrust out and your head looking directly ahead. Now tense your abdominal wall and drop down and back with your glutes to activate the movement, maintaining an upright torso position. Go down until your thighs are parallel with the floor. To avoid excess strain on the knees, don't go down any further. In the bottom squat position, your lower legs should be almost vertical to the floor. Push through your heels as you return to the starting position.

Because squats include an aerobic component, it's vital that you use proper breathing technique. If you don't you may start to feel light headed after a few repetitions. As you lower yourself breathe in deeply. Then on the way back up

Exercise 2: **Farmer's Walk**

Prime Mover: Quadriceps

Grab hold of a pair of dumbbells nd hold them at arms' length. Now take an exaggerated step forward so that your lead leg cones down to a parallel floor position and your trailing knee just touches the floor. Push through the front thigh to step out of this lunge position and into the next exaggerated step. Continue for the prescribed number of steps (reps). Then turn around and return to the start position.

Exercise 3: **Deadlift**

Prime Mover: Upper Back

Use extreme caution with the deadlift. This is a compound movement. It's always important to nail the form on a movement, but it is doubly important with deadlift. Avoid injury! Use no weight or light weights until you have the movement mastered!

Load a barbell and set it on the floor. Squat in front of it with your feet shoulder width apart. Grab it overhead with your hands just outside your legs, your shoulders over or just behind the bar, your arms straight and your back flat or slightly arched. Simple as it sounds, all you really do is stand up. The key is to push with your heels and pull the weight to your body as you stand. Pause with the weight, but don't lean back, then slowly return to the starting position.

Pause with the weight on the floor and reset your body over the bar. You defeat the purpose of the dead-lift if you use momentum to knock out the reps.

Exercise 4: **Lying Leg Curl**

Prime Mover; Hamstrings

Lie on the leg curl machine, hooking your feet under the leg curl bar. Drop your chest down flat against the bench but keep your head up and your back arched slightly (you will be in the "Sphinx" position). Curl the bar up as high as it will go. If you can't get it up all the way, decrease the weight. Leg curls are only effective when done with correct form. It's the tension in the hamstrings that counts, not the weight.

Exercise 5: **Standing Calf Raise**

Prime Mover: Soleus

Position yourself under a standing calf rise machine, with your shoulders resting on the shoulder pads. Place your toes on the edge of the foot plate and stand to an upright position. Keeping your knees locked throughout the movement, raise up on your toes to fully extend your calves. Hold at the top position for a slow count of three. Now, without bending your knees, lower to stretch your calves downward.

Exercise 6: **Reverse Crunch**

Prime Mover: Lower Abdominals

Lie with your arms at your sides. Hold your legs off the floor with your knees bent at a 90-degree angle so that your thighs point straight up and your lower legs point straight ahead, parallel to the floor. Crunch your pelvis towards your rib cage. Your tail bone should rise 2 to 3 inches off the floor as your knees move towards your chin. Pause, then slowly return to the starting position.

Exercise 7: **Plank**

Prime Mover: Upper Abdominals

Get into a modified push up position with your weight on your forearms and toes. Your body should form a straight line from head to heels (don't let your back sag). Pull you abs in as far as you can, and hold this position for 60 seconds, breathing steadily. If you can't get to 60 seconds in one go, break it up into 3 sets of 20 seconds and work up to the 60 second goal.

UPPER BODY: Workout B *New Exercises*

Exercise 2: **Lat Pull-Downs**

Prime Mover: Latissimus dorsi

Take a wide grip on a lat pull-down bar with a false overhand grip (thumb on the same side as your fingers). Keep your arms straight and your torso upright or leaning slightly back. Pull your shoulder blades together to bring the weight down. At the same time stick your chest out. Pull the bar to meet your chest. Pause with the bar 1 to 2 inches off your chest, then slowly let it rise to the starting position. Keep your chest out throughout the movement.

Exercise 4: **Incline Dumbbell Flies**

Prime Mover: Upper pectorals

Lie on a bench that is inclined to 30 degrees. Hold a pair of dumbbells in an overhand grip over your mid-pec region, with your arms straight up. Make sure that your feet are firmly planted on the floor. Maintaining a slight bend in your elbows, lower the dumbbells down and back until your upper arms are parallel to the floor and in line with your ears. Then use your chest to pull the weights back up to the starting position, retracing the same route in reverse. Keep your shoulder blades pinched back towards each other throughout, and flex your pecs at the top of the movement.

Exercise 6: **Side Lateral Raises**

Prime Mover: Deltoids

Hold two dumbbells, one in each hand, at your sides, palms facing your sides. Your feet should be shoulder width apart with your knees slightly bent. Tense your core as you raise the weights to shoulder level (no higher).

While you are lifting the weights out to the side, pretend that, instead of dumbbells, you have pitchers of water in your hands and that you are going to water some plants up at shoulder level. Allow your elbows to bend and your forearms to drift slightly forward. As you reach the top of the movement, rotate your shoulders forward so that the front plates of the dumbbells are slightly lower than the rear plates - just as if you were pouring water. This will cause you to raise your elbows slightly. The rotation needs to come from your shoulders, not your wrists or arms.

The pouring motion positions the lateral deltoid to take the brunt of the strain. If you don't 'pour', the front deltoid helps out too much, decreasing the efficiency of the exercise.

Exercise 7: **Triceps Pushdown**

Prime Mover: Triceps

Stand a foot or so away from the pulley on a triceps pushdown machine, holding the bar so that the cable angles slightly away from you. Your triceps are strongest about two thirds of the way through the movement and starting in this position adjusts the resistance curve to more closely match the triceps' strength curve.

Press the bar down in as wide a semi-circle as possible. Don't let your elbows drift back. This shortens the path the bar travels and decreases the amount of work done, limiting the effectiveness of the exercise. As you press, keep your wrists straight and your shoulders down.

Allowing the wrists to bend back increases the tendency to push straight down on the bar, instead of pressing it in a semi-circle. At the bottom of the motion, your elbows should be one or two inches in front of you, and your forearms should be parallel. Reverse the motion to raise the bar. Allow the bar to come up until it's even with your chin.

Exercise 8: **Incline Dumbbell Curls**

Prime Mover: Biceps

Set an incline bar at a 75-degree angle. Grasp two dumbbells with an underhand grip, straight down at arm's length. Curl the weights towards your shoulders. Stop and squeeze when the dumbbells are 6 to 8 inches in front of your shoulders. Hold the contraction, squeezing tight, for 2 seconds. Now, slowly return the dumbbells to the starting position. Be sure to resist gravity during the negative part of the movement.

LOWER BODY: Workout B *New Exercises*

Exercise 2: **Leg Press**

Prime Mover: Quadriceps

Sit back in the leg press station with your back against the pad and your feet shoulder width apart on the foot plate. Adjust the seat so that your knees are bent slightly more than 90 degrees. Now push the weight until your knees are straight but not locked. Keep your back flat and your neck straight. Pause, then return to the start position.

Do not allow your knees to buckle inward throughout this movement. Make sure to also avoid the temptation to place your hands on your knees to help push the weight. Keep your hands firmly gripping the handles throughout the movement. You should also focus your energy into your heels rather than the balls of your feet.

Exercise 5: **Kneeling Cable Crunch**

Prime Mover: Rectus abdominis

Attach a rope handle to a high pulley on a cable machine. Face the machine, grab the rope and kneel in front of the weight stack. Hold the ropes at the sides of your face with your elbows pointing straight down to the floor.

Crunch your rib cage towards your pelvis without moving any other part of your lower body from its original position. Pause when your elbows approach your knees, then slowly return to the starting position.

Exercise 6: **Prone Superman**

Prime Mover: Erector Spinae

Lie face down with your legs straight and your arms stretched straight in front of you, with your hands on the floor. Lift your arms, head, chest and lower legs off the floor simultaneously. Hold this position for 5 seconds, keeping your head and neck at the same height as your shoulders, throughout the movement. Return to the starting position.

Phase Three Exercises

New exercises . . .

Close Grip Bench Press

Prime Mover: Triceps

Position yourself on a bench press station as if you were about to perform the standard barbell bench press. The difference is in your hand spacing. The closer your hands are together, the more the focus of the exercise switches to your triceps. The ideal hand spacing is about six inches apart. Press the bar down to your sternum and push back in an arcing toward your upper chest. Consciously think about preventing the elbows from flaring out as you do this movement.

Face Pulls

Prime Mover: Trapezius

Stand in front of a high pulley machine with a rope handle. Take a hold of the handles with an overhand grip and stand with arms extended. Pull back so that the rope comes to your forward. As you come back, squeeze your shoulder blades together and think about contracting the muscles of the trapezius. Your elbows should come back and out with each repetition.

Dad Fitness Opportunities

In the first chapter of the book, the idea of dad as a role model when it comes to fitness and health is a powerful message for kids of all ages was highlighted. Not only does it show the value of being physically fit for your kids, but it starts them out on a pattern of behavior that will carry through with them as a basis for how they will live their life when they are out and on their own. A 2014 report from Iowa State University observed, "children and adolescents mirror the trends of their adult counterparts such that overweight children become overweight adults. Current literature reports parental obesity as one of the most powerful predictors of childhood obesity likely resulting from a combination of shared genes, habits, and environment." [134] Similarly, in the book *Growing Up Healthy: Protecting Your Child from Diseases Now Through Adulthood*, fitness expert and martial arts master Beth Ann Bielat reminds parents, "The more physically fit your children are at any age, the healthier they are at all ages. By getting your kids up and moving each day, you'll be giving them one of the greatest gifts in life – physical fitness, which will help to ensure quality of life and longevity". [135]

While going to the gym or "box" is important, and it will be essential if building lean body mass is your goal, that doesn't mean that fun activities and things with the kids can not be a part of your fitness routine.

Kids of all ages can and do enjoy doing things with their fathers. Moreover, time spent by children with their fathers provides a uniquely invaluable contribution to their development and well-being. Two studies, one from 1995 and another from 1999 confirmed "that the amount of time spent with fathers and the amount of emotional support obtained from fathers were associated with less depression, higher self-esteem, higher life satisfaction, and less delinquency" in their children. [136] By modeling a healthy lifestyle and bringing your children along with you, you are delivering a powerful, lifelong message to them. You are telling them, "I see in you a strong, vibrant, and eminently capable person. I know that you are that person. I respect you. I believe in you. I love you." As NCAA champion basketball coach Jim Valvano recounted, "My father gave me the greatest gift anyone could give another person, he believed in me".

There is something that can be done at any age; you may just have to become a bit creative. For infants and toddlers, consider a jogging stroller. These are not at all like typical strollers, but they will provide a safe, comfortable ride for the child as well as being ergonomically designed to make it comfortable for the jogger as well. Accomplish some of your cardio outside pushing your child along with you in the jogger. You could stop at various points along the way and accomplish some resistance training with your child parked right next to you. Many neighborhood parks have fitness installations that allow you to do things like pull-ups and dips. Alternatively, you could do pull-ups from tree branches (it goes without saying, be safe and smart about activities like this). Some great, compact products available at a reasonable price that can serve as go-anywhere pieces of fitness equipment are a jump rope, a collapsible ab roller, and the "Lifeline Jungle Gym XT" (which is similar to TRX straps but significantly less expensive).

Children that are a bit older can always bike alongside their dad, which is a great way to get in some quality time. Kids can even do HIIT training geared to their level. By taking the competitiveness out of the activity and simply keeping it as a personal-best type of activity, everyone can spend some time together. Go to the local American football field or soccer pitch and do interval training with your kids or run the stairs at a local stadium or park. Younger kids can do shorter intervals while Dads and teens can go longer.

Playing sports with kids and finding new workout opportunities that are family friendly is also an ideal way to spend time together. Try rock climbing, hiking, kayaking or other types of sports to not only increase your workout options, but also to help your children understand how fitness is an important part of being in the shape you want to be able to enjoy life.

Another option to consider is to set up a small home gym in your house. Free weights and a bench. If you have a spare room, add a power cage. A universal barbell and plates make a great addition as well.

Plateaus and Tracking Performance

In the first century AD, the Roman philosopher and statesman Seneca said it best, "Our plans miscarry because they have no aim. When a man does not know what harbour he is making for, no wind is the right wind." [137] It is the same with fitness; if you do not have goals and you do not measure progress, it can become impossible to see progress once the initial big weight loss occurs. To add to this, there are times when you will have plateaus, so seeing where you have come from and where you are going is important as a mental motivator.

Plateaus are part of the game with a long-term fitness lifestyle. If you persist long enough, you are going to deal with them. If you get stuck in a plateau for too long, though, motivation can wane significantly. You could even give up completely on your quest to get ripped.

The reason is because progress is essential to motivation. When progress stalls, the human psyche can flounder. Tony Robbins, the master of self-development, explains, "If you want to have ongoing joy and fulfillment in your life, the secret is just one word – progress. Progress equals happiness. While achievements and material things may excite you for the moment, the only thing that's going to make you happy long-term is knowing that you're making progress. To do this, you must remember: While change is automatic – progress is not. Progress results from actively and consciously choosing to create a life you love; a life where you can't wait to jump out of bed in the morning because you are growing, contributing, impacting and serving." [138]

Recognizing plateaus when they do occur and understanding why they are occurring is the best solution to pushing beyond them. Plateaus can occur at any time in a training routine. Plateaus are best defined as true flat spots or regressions in your weight loss and muscle-building plan.

But before identifying a flat spot or a regression as a true plateau, you need to assess the situation. Are you in "the dip" or are you in a true plateau? The dip is a reference to the book by author and entrepreneur Seth Godin by the same name. Mr. Godin explains that when you first start almost anything, the progress is rapid: in fitness, at first, pounds drop off easily, inches disappear from your waist, and strength explodes. "And then the Dip happens. The Dip is the long slog between starting and mastery." Progress slows down. What was new now seems monotonous. This is the point at which many people give up and quit. [139]

Ask yourself, especially if you are relatively new to fitness: am I in a true plateau or am in the dip? If you are in the dip, understand that if you truly want to get that ripped body (and you definitely can): "The people who set out to make it through the Dip—the people who invest the time and the energy and the effort to power through the Dip ... instead of moving on to the next thing, instead of doing slightly above average and settling for what they've got, they embrace the challenge. For whatever reason, they refuse to abandon the quest and they push through the Dip all the way to the next level." [140]

Realize that you cannot continue to lose an inch every two weeks from your waist, you cannot drop ten pounds every month, you cannot continue to add ten pounds per week to your incline press 1RM. If that were true, you would eventually shrivel away to nothing and you could incline press 1000 pounds within two or three years. Eventually, that kind of progress has to slow down. But there are also other kinds of progress to make in your fitness journey from which you can draw inspiration and motivation.

Beyond the dip, there are several reasons that plateaus will happen on the way to getting ripped. One of the most common is overtraining and failing to build in enough recovery time. Your body requires rest. Your central nervous system (CNS) requires rest.

For a long time, I thought only my muscles were subject to fatigue as a result of my workouts. Wrong. The CNS is an integral component to putting up weight at high intensity and/or high volume. In situations when, for example, you struggle with all your might to complete that last repetition or when you are lifting your maximum load, you can feel the stress on your muscles.

What many people do not realize, though, is that the CNS is working just as hard or harder to fire the neurons and maintain the intensity required to power through your lifts. The CNS can get worn out. While muscles can recover in a couple of days from an intense workout, the CNS can take longer in some cases. "CNS fatigue has been linked to a host of neurochemical changes that may have time courses longer than that of muscle metabolic fatigue ... Hence even if a muscle is metabolically recovered, the nervous system may not be capable of recruiting high-threshold fibers.". [141]

One of the reasons why caffeine is an ingredient in so many pre-workout "stacks" and why it is recognized as a performance-enhancer is not because it stimulates the muscles, but because it stimulates the CNS: "Recent findings suggest that low doses of caffeine exert significant ergogenic effects by directly affecting the central nervous system during exercise. Caffeine can cross the blood–brain barrier and antagonize the effects of adenosine, resulting in higher concentrations of stimulatory neurotransmitters. These new data strengthen the case for using low doses of caffeine during training." [142]

Falling victim to overtraining may mean you have not yet learned how to listen effectively to your body's subtle (and sometimes not-so-subtle) nuances and have been pushing heavy training even on days when you were already fatigued coming into the gym. It may be time for a rest day (or two or three days). Experiment with taking strategic time away from the gym. Or it may be worthwhile to try adjusting your workout and doing lighter weights for a day (or a week), and pushing harder again when you feel recovered.

Stress is another common reason for plateaus. Stress (both good stress and bad stress) from work, family, relationships, and our various commitments can constrain our time and further tax our CNS. When people are under stress they tend to develop poor sleep hygiene and/or have trouble sleeping. Sleep quality is a critical, perhaps *the* critical, input to our overall well-being. If you are not sleeping well, you are going to have issues. According to sleep medicine specialist and former US Navy SEAL, Dr. Kirk Parsley, sleep is "the LAST thing you should be skimping on. In my estimation, if you are going to chronically ignore any of the 4 pillars of health (Sleep, Nutrition, Exercise, Stress control), make sleep your last choice to ignore. Am I saying eat doughnuts for breakfast instead of sleeping 6 hours and eating kale for breakfast? Yes I am. Am I saying get 8 hours of sleep every night, even if that means you will no longer have time to exercise? Yes I am.
Am I saying give up your meditation, mindfulness, breathing techniques before giving up sleep? Yes I am. The truth is that NOTHING will break you faster than inadequate or low quality sleep. There is a reason sleep deprivation is used to break down people for interrogation. The reason is because it works! Fast!" [143]

Stress can drain our energy as much as, or more than, training does. Worry and anxiety fire up the brain with electrical activity. That requires energy. If you have chronic problems with stress and anxiety, there are a range of ways to address it from meditation to individual or group therapy. A spiritual practice is profoundly helpful in stress management.

Obviously, diet is also a fundamental component of our overall health. Times of stress are a setup for poor food choices and consuming an excess of calories. Not all types of foods are the same, even with the same caloric content. Choosing highly processed, fatty, high-carbohydrate and high-sugar foods will have an impact on your metabolism and your ability to fuel cells for muscle growth and repair. You can work out all day long with the best form and do everything right in the gym, but if your diet is off, you will not succeed long-term.

Fitness Trackers and Other Helpful Tools

As you begin your fitness journey and begin stepping down the road toward getting ripped, it is highly recommended that you document your performance. Doing this will provide you with objective information as to your progress (or lack thereof). Documenting your performance can be as simple as measuring your waist once a week with a measuring tape to as technologically advanced as getting regular DEXA body composition scans and utilizing a variety of wi-fi or Bluetooth-enabled fitness trackers. A 2017 review article from the journal *Frontiers in Public Health* explained, "The use of technology, including fitness trackers and smartphone apps, show a great deal of promise for measuring and encouraging physical activity". [144]

Benchmarking and documenting markers of health is easier now than ever before, with fitness trackers, heart rate monitors, calorie and nutrition tracking mobile apps, wi-fi enabled body weight and body composition scales, and equipment that provides instant information as to the effectiveness of your routine. Seeing those numbers improve and setting objective, measurable goals and then achieving them is a great form of motivation for your initial fitness plans as well as a long term way to keep yourself on track and in the program.

By far one of the least expensive and simplest ways to assess your overall health is by computing your waist-to-height ratio. The only equipment you need is a tape measure (and perhaps a calculator). About two-and-a-half years ago, when I was struggling to shed my "dad bod", I went to see my primary care physician, Dr Ted Naiman of BurnFatNotSugar.com to discuss a battery of routine blood tests.

I was very confused by what all of the different results meant and was talking them over with Dr. Naiman. In the course of that conversation, I casually mentioned my waist size at the time. I did not think it was a big deal. Dr Naiman immediately stopped the conversation and said, "Whoa! Hold on. What did you say your waist size was?" You see, with clothes on, I did not look particularly chunky compared to the ever-fattening population of American men my age.

I was what you call "TOFI" (Thin Outside, Fat Inside) or "skinny fat". TOFI is an extremely unhealthy condition characterized by an excess buildup of visceral fat in the abdominal trunk. A 2013 study, for example, found that TOFI patients had "the highest risk of mortality". [145]

I repeated my waist size to him. In reply, he said, "We can just stop talking about all of these blood test results. Your waist size tells me all I need to know. It's a way more accurate marker of overall health than this blood test. The ideal waist size for a man is 45% of his height". I did some quick math in my head and realized I was far over 45%. I had a lot of work to do.

Repeated studies have determined that waist-to-height ratio correlates positively with BMI, total cholesterol, blood pressure, and fasting blood glucose (a critical health marker) and is a more effective tool for screening for cardiovascular disease, stroke risk, and diabetes than BMI and waist circumference. Different studies have determined that the ideal waist-to-height ratio ranges from .45 to .5 for men. [146] An important point to be aware of when measuring your waist is that your waist circumference is

NOT the same thing as your pants size. Measure your waist around your belly button.

Another measurement that is cheap and easy to perform is your waist-to-chest ratio. Studies have found that a ratio of .6 with a mesomorphic body shape is considered ideally attractive by women. Think of a mesomorph body shape as the in-between body shape. An ectomorph is a slender male body shape and an endomorph is a burlier male body shape. Another study found that the single most unattractive male body feature to women is a protruding abdomen. [147] So, men, both in terms of health and longevity, and in terms of your physical attractiveness, you need to lose the gut.

The next tracking tool on the list is some sort of calorie-tracking app. Personally, I use MyFitnessPal. It is free and simple to use. It has an extensive database of foods available via an internet connection so that I only need to spend a couple of seconds inputting my meals into the app. In the rare instances when a food does not instantly appear in their database when I input it, MyFitnessPal has a barcode-scanning feature that retrieves the information for me. Not only does MyFitnessPal allow me to monitor my calorie intake, but it also gives me awareness of all of my macros (carbohydrates, proteins, and fats) along with cholesterol, vitamins, and minerals. If you are going to lose fat, you must develop a daily caloric deficit. MyFitnessPal makes me very cognizant of where I stand every day with respect to my calorie balance. MyFitnessPal's web site will allow you to link all of your fitness apps and trackers in one central dashboard.

I also highly recommend tracking workouts in some way. I use a Microsoft Excel spreadsheet on my phone as a workout tracker. I record all of my repetitions, weights, and where I am forced to rest and fail during sets. However, you can use old-school pen and paper or download a fitness-tracking app for your phone.

Continuous fitness trackers come in all different styles and at all different prices. FitBit and Garmin are two popular and well-known brands along with the Apple Watch. Most of the newer models automatically track heart rate, steps, and sleep. Ideally, invest in a quality tracker that recognizes different types of workouts and provides the information you need for your plan. Some of the top trackers allow for interval training, cardio workouts and for customized training programs. They can be used to track your activities, calories burned, food intake, sleep and other customized tracking options. An excellent, free web site to read extensive reviews of a wide variety of fitness technology gear is DCRainmaker.com.

I use a Garmin triathlon type of watch all day and pair it with a chest strap during workouts. It tracks and stores my heart rate during all of my resistance training workouts. During my cardio running sessions, it tracks my cadence, left-right balance, ground contact time, vertical height, and several other measures that allow me to analyze my "running dynamics". To me, it has become an indispensable part of my workout ecosystem. My Garmin watch also sync's automatically with MyFitnessPal so I can compare my calories burned during the day with my calories consumed.

Using a fitness tracker in combination with a heart rate monitor is a great way to get a very specific reading throughout your workout of where you are versus where you need to be. You can plot your resting heart rate and fat burning zone and monitor your workout to stay in the fat burning zone and maximize results. Heart rate information is extremely useful during all kinds of workouts.

Next up: look for a good scale, which is ideally WiFi-enabled. Most of these types of scales can be linked to your fitness tracker and your food logs. I use a Nokia BodyCardio scale that measures my body composition and cardiovascular health in addition to my weight. It also syncs automatically with MyFitnessPal and Garmin. I can view my progress on the Nokia app on my phone which graphs all of my measurements over time. That is extremely motivating information. If I am doing well, I am encouraged. If I am beginning to regress, I immediately see it and take action.

An additional item to track that can be useful is blood glucose. This reading is performed via a quick and virtually painless finger prick. It uses the same equipment diabetics use to monitor their blood glucose. You can pick up a glucose monitor and some test strips for less than $30 (US) online. In my opinion, the most useful measurement is fasting blood glucose (FBG), as opposed to "postprandial" (after eating) blood glucose. FBG is typically read in the morning after not eating for the past eight to twelve hours. "Higher-than-optimum blood glucose is a leading cause of cardiovascular mortality in most world regions", [148] and "elevated fasting [blood] glucose levels and a diagnosis of diabetes are independent risk factors for several major cancers, and the risk tends to increase with an increased level of fasting [blood] glucose". [149] In fact, Alzheimer's disease is referred to by many specialists as "Diabetes Type 3" for its association with poor glucose control. A 2008 study stated, "impaired fasting glucose occur[s] significantly more frequently in [Alzheimer's disease] than in non-[Alzheimer's disease] controls". [150] And a 2018 report in the journal *Diabetologia* established a link between glucose levels and cognitive decline as we age. The report explained, glucose "levels were linearly associated with subsequent cognitive decline in memory and executive function..." [151]

Finally, I highly recommend obtaining a DEXA body composition scan as you begin your fitness program. DEXA stands for dual-energy X-ray absorptiometry. It is the most accurate way to measure your body composition that is widely available at a reasonable price (MRI and ultrasound are more accurate but not easily available and are expensive). DEXA measures the amount of fat in different "compartments" of your body: trunk, left and right arms, left and right legs, and even your head. It also tells you how much lean mass you have. In addition, some DEXA providers will supply you with your own individualized resting metabolic rate (RMR), which is extremely valuable in terms of computing the amount of calories you require per day. Most importantly, though, is the ability to determine how much fat you have in your "trunk" – your abdominal area. Visceral fat in this area is far more dangerous than in other areas of your body. The entire process takes about 30-45 minutes to complete and is painless. Follow up your initial DEXA scan with subsequent scans on a fairly regular basis. How often is up to you: two to three times per year should be more than adequate.

3. Nutrition And Supplements

Diet Comes First

Attempting to decipher the swirl of often conflicting information and "bro science" that orbits around diet and nutrition in the world of gaining muscle and losing fat can take on the appearance of a hopeless, quixotic task. Which diet should you choose in the seemingly endless parade of fad diets: paleo, intermittent fasting, ketogenic, Atkins, the Zone, South Beach, Mediterranean, detox, raw food, alkaline, blood-type?

My advice for anyone who wants to get fit and stay that way at any time in their life, but especially as they enter into middle age and older, is to pick the low-hanging fruit first. Do not attempt to get into the weeds of diet science until you have taken care of the basics. That will cover 90% of your bases.

In the case of diet and supplements, the easy-to-reach low-hanging fruit is to concentrate the vast majority of your diet on eating healthy whole foods, avoiding processed foods as much as possible. A good rule of thumb to use is: if the food was manufactured in a factory, try to avoid it. A 2012 Canadian study put it this way, "any substantial improvement of the diet would involve much lower consumption of ultra-processed products and much higher consumption of meals and dishes prepared from minimally processed foods and processed culinary ingredients." [152]

Before you spend substantial sums of money on diet programs of any sort, expensive supplements, or workout equipment, you can make tremendous improvements in your health and fitness by simply eating whole, minimally processed foods. If you can take this one gigantic step, you will be well on your way to the shredded body you want.

You can spend hours upon hours at the gym, but if your diet is not on track, you are largely wasting your time if you want to get ripped. As Dr. Todd Astorino, an exercise scientist at the University of California, San Marcos explained in a *Prevention* magazine piece, "Even if you don't exercise, if you ate really well you could probably look like an athlete and be fairly healthy. But if your diet is poor, no amount of exercise will make up for that." [153]

Think about it this way, 60 minutes of an intense resistance training session at the gym burns about 600 calories for a 180 pound man. If you slow-roll the resistance workout, you may only burn as little as 200 calories. 30 minutes of super-intense, maximum effort running burns about 650 calories. 30 minutes of moderate-paced running burns around 350 calories.

Now for the reality check: eat one Big Mac (540 calories) and you nearly obliterated almost the entire benefit of a hard, hour-long workout. If your workout was not intense, you would have had to spend nearly three hours in the gym to compensate for one Big Mac. How long does it take you to eat a Big Mac?

Add medium fries (340 calories) and a medium Coke (220 calories), and you are far behind even after an intense workout. [154] Prefer Starbucks? Have a chicken sausage and bacon biscuit sandwich (450 calories) along with a grande Chai Crème Frappuccino® Blended Crème drink (210 calories) and once again, you have more than negated the calorie-burning impact of your hard workout. Adding whipped cream to that drink piles on 110 more calories, putting you that much further into the hole. [155]

Those examples, by the way, only take into consideration the caloric energy balance impact of an undisciplined diet. Eating unhealthy, processed foods also has a wide range of other negative effects on your body like, for example, contributing to insulin resistance which, in turn, over time often leads to type 2 diabetes. Those effects, many would argue, are more harmful than the excess calories. Is it worth it?

To give you an idea of what is possible with diet and minimal exercise alone, look at the screen shot below from my weight tracking app. That screen shot is my body weight tracked over a period of about three months (the volatile ups and downs are simply reflective of how much weight varies during the course of a day due to water weight, food ingestion, etc). When I began my transformation out of "dad bod" territory, I was so out of shape, I could not even tolerate simple resistance sessions. I had tried several times to begin resistance training again at the intensity level I had previously been able to maintain and had promptly torn various muscles three separate times. Each incidence set me back weeks.

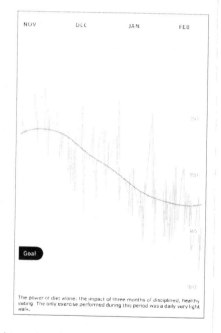

The power of diet alone: the impact of three months of disciplined, healthy eating. The only exercise performed during this period was a daily very light walk.

I knew I had to do something different. I consulted a functional medicine practitioner. He informed me that my approach to diet was essentially all wrong. At the time, I ate what I thought was a "healthy" diet. It turns out, unbeknownst to me, I had bought into the lies of the Big Food lobby. I took pride in my consumption of foods like organic vegetable and fruit smoothies, Clif Bars and "low fat" yogurt. I never really thought about caloric balance very much. I had no idea what insulin resistance was.

The functional medicine expert told me to immediately stop consuming almost everything I had been consuming, especially the smoothies I was so proud of. "But I thought they were healthy", I protested. In reply, he explained, "No, no, no. When you blend fruit and vegetables up, you take them out of their natural form. You separate them from their fiber. When you do that, you create a huge blood sugar spike followed shortly after by a huge insulin spike. He advised me to start taking my blood sugar readings (and he was right, my blood sugar did surge after smoothies). He told me to make it a point to eat huge serving-bowl size portions of salad every day. He also emphasized the importance of healthy fats from grass-fed beef, wild-caught seafood, and pasture-raised poultry or pork. Finally, he explained that I should also get plenty of healthy fats from sources like organic, cold-pressed, extra-virgin olive oil, organic coconut oil, and medium-chain triglyceride (MCT) oil.

As noted above, he advised me to begin checking my blood glucose level. I was horrified to discover that my fasting blood glucose level had been creeping up over the years (with no warning from my traditional insurance-controlled doctor) to an almost pre-diabetic level. I also discovered that my blood glucose level shot skyward after eating certain foods and rose precipitously during stressful periods. Again, elevated fasting blood glucose levels are a strong indicator of health risk but so is a volatile blood glucose level. A 2011 meta-analysis explained, "All studies reported a statistically significant association between mortality and at least one glucose variability indicator." [156]

What you see in the above screen shot is the impact of changing my diet from an undisciplined regimen of what I thought was healthy food to a disciplined diet recommended by the functional health practitioner. I began intermittent fasting at about the midway point of the period depicted in the screen shot. What is not shown on that graph is that my waist size also shrank by approximately three inches and my blood glucose readings began trending down toward normal ranges. The only exercise performed during that course of time was light walking nearly every day. That, to me, is a compelling example of the power of diet.

As an additional note, I had a DEXA scan performed before beginning my "dad bod" journey and another performed a few months after the period illustrated in the above screen shot from my weight tracking app. You can see the results from my DEXA scans, side-by-side, in the graphic below. During that time, I lost nearly a full gallon of fat (six pounds) from my abdominal area and gained nearly six pounds of muscle. I had started light resistance training again shortly before taking the second DEXA scan, but the majority of those results can be attributed to diet and light walking alone.

	Fat Mass (lbs)	Lean Mass (lbs)		Fat Mass (lbs)	Lean Mass (lbs)
L. Arm	1.7	10.4	L. Arm	1.4	11.0
R. Arm	2.0	11.4	R. Arm	1.5	11.7
Trunk	18.1	66.5	Trunk	12.1	68.9
L Leg	7.7	23.2	L Leg	5.9	24.4
R Leg	7.9	23.6	R Leg	5.7	24.5
Subtotal	37.4	135.1	Subtotal	26.5	140.6
Head	2.5	7.7	Head	2.6	7.9
Total	**39.9**	142.8	**Total**	**29.0**	148.4
Android	3.3	0.0	Android	2.0	0.0
Gynoid	8.2	0.0	Gynoid	5.9	0.0

Results of DEXA scans six months apart after a radical change in diet with very little exercise: a loss of six pounds of fat from the trunk/abdominal area (nearly a full gallon) and a gain of almost six pounds of muscle.

Th

e bottom line is diet is critical to your success toward achieving a ripped body. Exercise is also necessary if you want to get ripped, but diet is foundational and needs to come first.

To recap, when looking for healthy foods, think natural and non-processed. If it comes in a box, can, or in a tray, it is probably processed. Think of eating meats, seafood, poultry, eggs, fresh vegetables, fresh fruits, dairy, legumes and whole grains. This is the subject for a different discussion, but realize that many health-conscious individuals entirely avoid certain types of foods like dairy, legumes, and grains. If you have access to it, grass-fed beef and dairy, wild-caught seafood, and pasture-raised poultry are highly preferred, healthier sources of meat. Likewise, organic, non-genetically-modified (non-GMO) produce is also a much better option than produce that has been sprayed with pesticides.

Calories matter. By avoiding processed, high-sugar, and high carbohydrate foods, you feel full faster and tend to eat less. At the same time, less processed foods from healthier source are richer in macro and micronutrients, which aid in reducing the urge to eat or to snack, as well as providing the fuel your body needs.

Protein

Hypertrophy is driven by a process called muscle protein synthesis (MPS). Proteins are the building block of life. A primary function of DNA, for instance, is to encode the instructions for building proteins. Proteins are critical not only for hypertrophy but for every aspect of life. Proteins are composed of amino acids. There are twenty different types of amino acids used by the human body. Nine of these types of amino acids are deemed "essential amino acids" (EAA's) because the human body cannot synthesize them. We must obtain EAA's from food. "Proteins possess an extremely important property: a protein spontaneously folds into a well-defined and elaborate three-dimensional structure that is dictated entirely by the sequence of amino acids along its chain." The loss of just one amino acid out of a chain of close to 1500 amino acids, for example in the case of cystic fibrosis, causes a life-threatening condition. [157]

In a muscle cell, or myofiber, its fundamental component is a myofibril. Myofibrils, in turn, are composed of structures constructed primarily from the proteins myosin and actin: "In muscle cells, thick filaments made up of myosin and thin filaments made up of actin compose structures called sarcomeres, which are the basic units of muscle contraction. The overlapping thick and thin filaments bind to each other and release, which allows the filaments to move relative to one another so that muscles can contract." [158]

Since myosin and actin are both proteins, and are absolutely fundamental to muscular function, it goes without saying that protein intake is critical to our muscular development. A 2012 study from *The Journal of Physiology* explained, "The anabolic [muscle building] effects of nutrition are principally driven by the transfer and incorporation of amino acids captured from dietary protein sources, into skeletal muscle proteins." [159] So, muscle protein synthesis is driven by amino acid availability. We provide our body with those amino acids by consuming protein.

But how much protein do we need?

In the world of bodybuilding and strength athletes, guidelines vary widely regarding how much protein is ideal for muscle synthesis and hypertrophy. There is a huge range of recommended daily protein intake. I have heard everything from .8 grams of protein per pound of body weight per day all the way up to two grams per pound of body weight. What is the right amount?

Let's look at the science. A 2011 study from the *British Journal of Nutrition* explained, "it appears that emerging dietary guidelines for protein are in the range of 1.2–1.6 [grams of protein per kilogram per day]. This level is greater than the [recommended daily allowance (RDA)], with the general recommendation that the RDA is a protein intake designed simply to alleviate deficiency." According to this study, the recommended daily protein intake works out to be approximately 100-130 grams of protein per day for a 180-pound guy. The *Journal* goes on to explain that what is critically important is the timing of the protein intake – protein should be consumed at most, two hours after completing a workout; preferably immediately afterward. Interestingly, the study also said, "The high quality protein dose that appears to maximally stimulate muscle protein synthesis is close to 20–25 g, above which protein synthesis is not additionally stimulated but increases in amino acid oxidation and urea synthesis may result." [160] According to this study, then, it is not productive and perhaps even counter-productive to slurp down more than 20-25 grams of protein in a single dose.

So that settles it right? Not necessarily. A 2013 analysis from the *International Journal of Sport Nutrition and Exercise Metabolism* specifically examined the protein requirements of athletes undergoing caloric restriction during weight training. That is exactly the circumstance anyone who is attempting to shed fat and gain muscle will often find themselves in. The study explained what makes this situation different than the situation of typical athletes: "Slight energy deficits increase protein requirements which are further increased with exercise ... Greater caloric restriction (1100kcal/day versus 550kcal/day) can lead to declines in anabolic hormones and decrements in performance ... Fast rates of weight loss in athletes with low body fat often results in [fat-free-mass] losses." [161] The researchers are making the point that when you are taking in less calories per day than you are expending, it creates a unique metabolic scenario that significantly drives up the body's need for protein.

The researchers in this study concluded that when a person is exercising and in a state of negative energy balance, a protein intake of 2.3-3.1 grams per kilogram of fat-free-mass per day is recommended to protect against the loss of lean mass. For example, I have about 155 pounds, or 70 kilograms, of fat-free-mass. When I am in a state of negative energy balance (which has lately been very often), according to this study, my protein intake should be in the range of 160-220 grams of protein per day. The study guides people who have lower body fat and would

110

like to stay that way toward the higher end of the range and people concerned mostly with performance toward the lower end of the range.

Okay, now we have an answer, right? Not really. Menno Henselmans, the highly respected fitness authority behind Bayesian Bodybuilding created a detailed rebuttal to the above study. Henselmans took issue with nearly every aspect of the study, concluding in the end, "There are quite a few relevant studies, even of strength trainees in a deficit, and not a single one of them has found statistically significant benefits of consuming more than 1.6 g/kg protein. Nor is there a notable trend towards benefits. In fact, 1 study found detrimental body composition effects of going higher in protein. This research converges with several other studies in untrained subjects, nitrogen balance research and the body's theoretical physiology to indicate that protein requirements are not higher in a deficit than when at maintenance or when bulking. So I tell most of my clients: make sure to consume 1.8 g/kg protein, but don't worry about having to need more. Instead, enjoy the extra carbs or fats!" [162] Using Menno Henselmans protein recommendations, a 180 pound man would need just under 150 grams of protein per day to gain all of the benefits.

What kinds of protein should we get? In general, the go-to source for meeting our protein needs should be whole foods. Meats are very high in protein. For example, one four-ounce serving of chicken breast contains just under 34 grams of protein. [163] A four-ounce serving of 90% lean grass-fed ground beef contains 22 grams of protein. [164] By the way, as an aside, the primary reason to eat grass-feed beef is not because it tastes better or to indulge in some sort of luxurious extravagance. Grass-fed beef is healthier. In the same way human beings did not evolve as a species eating corn chips and slurping high fructose corn syrup, cattle did not evolve consuming corn or other grains. A 2010 review article from the *BMC Nutrition Journal* expounds, "Research spanning three decades supports the argument that grass-fed beef (on a [gram for gram] basis) has a more desirable [saturated fatty acid] lipid profile ... as compared to grain-fed beef. Grass-fed beef is also higher in total [conjugated linoleic acid] isomers ... Grass-fed beef is also higher in precursors for Vitamin A and E and cancer fighting antioxidants ... as compared to grain-fed contemporaries. Grass-fed beef also tends to be lower in overall fat content ..." [165]

When whole foods are not an option, whey protein is an excellent alternative for fulfilling protein requirements. Whey protein can be packed in zip-loc bags for travel (DO NOT make the mistake I did, though, and bring a big zip-loc bag full of protein powder with you to a foreign country! Customs gets very nervous. After being held up for two hours by border agents testing my protein powder with a spectrometer and the threat of an overseas prison sentence, I was finally cleared to proceed).

Whey protein is one of the most extensively studied supplements. Contrary to myth, whey protein has not been shown to harm the kidneys or liver, unless there is existing kidney or liver dysfunction. [166] In that case, make sure you consult your doctor before increasing your protein intake.

One final point: when consuming protein for hypertrophy, it is important to consider the leucine content of the protein source. Leucine is an EAA and it is also a branched chain amino acid. Remember, since it is an EAA, the human body cannot produce it. We must obtain it from our diet. Studies have determined that a serving dose of 3-4 grams of leucine stimulates maximum MPS. "Leucine alone appears to be nearly as effective in stimulating protein synthesis as when all branched chain amino acids (BCAAs) are consumed." [167]

To provide some perspective on the power of proteins, particularly leucine, to promote muscle growth, researchers conducted an eight-week study with participants performing the same workout regimen. One group was supplemented with whey protein and leucine while the other group consumed a placebo. After eight weeks, the supplemented group all showed "significant" performance increases in bench press and push-ups and "significant" increases in "total mass, fat-free mass, and lean body mass". The control group showed no change in any of those measures. [168]

Diet Options

When it comes to following a specific type of diet, there are many options. For guys who want to focus on weight loss and muscle growth, there are a few diets that get more attention than others.

Ketogenic Diet

"Ketogenesis" is an enormous buzzword lately within the fitness and functional health world. According to some, it would seem that ketogenesis is the holy grail of nutrition – a panacea for all that ails you. A ketogenic diet is typically synonymous with a low-carb, high-fat (LCHF) diet. "Ketogenesis" refers to the process that occurs when fatty acids are broken down within the liver into a group of substances knows as "ketone bodies". The names of these ketone bodies are acetone, beta-hydroxybutyrate, and acetoacetate. Ketone bodies are typically only produced when the body's normal fuel source, carbohydrates (or glucose), is "so scarce that energy must be obtained from the breaking down of fatty acids." [169] In other words, you are burning fat for fuel, instead of glucose.

The benefits of a ketogenic diet are touted as burning "more fat for fuel at a given intensity", obtaining "a more stable blood sugar", recovering "faster from your workouts – keto is anti-inflammatory", and attaining "a higher degree of mental clarity". [170] In general, to get into ketosis, "a carbohydrate intake below 50 [grams] is required".[171] However, many ketogenic diet advocates suggest a target of 20 grams of carbohydrates per day or less. The vast majority of calories consumed in a ketogenic diet come from healthy fats. MCT and coconut oil, for example, are hot commodities within the ketogenic community.

When ketone bodies are being produced, a person is said to be in a state of "ketosis". Ketone bodies can be used by the body for energy in lieu of the body's normal energy source, glucose. Since ketone bodies are down-regulated from stored body fat, ketosis generally results in a relatively rapid loss of fat.

In that sense, in terms of "getting ripped", a ketogenic diet can be a great place to start if you have a significant amount of stored body fat to lose. Realize, however, that if you begin a ketogenic diet, you will likely feel sluggish and perhaps even ill for up to the first several weeks since most people's metabolisms are not adapted to burning ketones. It takes the body a period of time to wake up that part of the metabolism. It is very much like when you first start lifting weights – your muscles are not adapted to the resistance. It takes time to catch up. This overall malaise when transitioning to a ketogenic diet is often referred to as "the keto flu". Symptoms can include: dizziness, brain fog, cramping, sore muscles, nausea, sugar cravings, stomach pain, among other similar symptoms. [172]

When I initially began my transition out of my "dad bod", I used a ketogenic diet and did lose a significant amount of weight and fat – at first. However, I am not using a ketogenic diet at the moment because I found that, in terms of building muscle, eating a diet higher in healthier carbohydrates is much more effective. As described by Krista Scott-Dixon, Ph.D. and Helen K. Kollias, Ph.D. at PrecisionNutrition.com, "Trying to build muscle while in ketosis is like stepping on the gas and the brake at the same time." [173]

This happens because a ketogenic diet depletes the body's glycogen stores, which are the fuel your muscles need. This means you will have less ability to maintain intensity in a workout, which in turn is not effective at building muscle tissue.

While there are some benefits to ketogenic dieting, especially if you have fat to shed, as a long-term solution for building muscle it may not be the best choice as a diet option. However, since the ketogenic diet so effectively sheds stored body fat in the initial stages of a body transformation program, I am including the Ripped Dad sample weekly meal plan for a ketogenic diet as a way to get you started on your journey toward achieving the ripped body you want. It includes delicious recipes, low in carbohydrates and high in healthy fats, designed to melt away body fat.

The *Ripped Dad* Sample Seven-Day Ketogenic Meal Plan

Monday

Breakfast	Lunch	Dinner
Avocado Baked Eggs	Quesadilla with Creamy Mushroom Dip	Pickled Salmon
Calories: 372 Fats: 32g Net Carbs: 6g Protein: 16g	Calories: 404 Fats: 43g Net Carbs: 2.4g Protein: 21g	Calories: 370 Fats: 4g Net Carbs: 7g Protein: 23g

Tuesday

Breakfast	Lunch	Dinner
Maple Flavored Pork Bake	Veal Picata	Bacon Chili Burgers
Calories: 405 Fats: 37g Net Carbs: 17g Protein: 1.9g	Calories: 325 Fats: 20g Net Carbs: 1g Protein: 32g	Calories: 485 Fats: 38g Net Carbs: 2g Protein: 31g

Wednesday

Breakfast	Lunch	Dinner
Avocado Tuna Melt Bites	Curried Chicken Salad	Orange Tequila Steak
Calories: 352 Fats: 36g Net Carbs: 5.5g Protein: 25g	Calories: 318 Fats: 24g Net Carbs: 3g Protein: 22g	Calories: 560 Fats: 46g Net Carbs: 5g Protein: 26g

Thursday

Breakfast	Lunch	Dinner
Avocado Baked Eggs	Tandoori Chicken	Smoky Marinated Steak
Calories: 372 Fats: 32g Net Carbs: 6g Protein: 16g	Calories: 503 Fats: 30g Net Carbs: 4g Protein: 52g	Calories: 276 Fats: 20g Net Carbs: 1g Protein: 23g

Friday

Breakfast	Lunch	Dinner
Breakfast Casserole	Quesadilla with Creamy Mushroom Dip	Pickled Salmon
Calories: 311 Fats: 32g Net Carbs: 5.8g Protein: 18g	Calories: 404 Fats: 43g Net Carbs: 2.4g Protein: 21g	Calories: 370 Fats: 4g Net Carbs: 7g Protein: 23g

Saturday

Breakfast	Lunch	Dinner
Maple Flavored Pork Bake	Veal Picata	Bacon Chili Burgers
Calories: 405 Fats: 37g Net Carbs: 17g Protein: 1.9g	Calories: 325 Fats: 20g Net Carbs: 1g Protein: 32g	Calories: 485 Fats: 38g Net Carbs: 2g Protein: 31g

Sunday

Breakfast	Lunch	Dinner
Avocado Tuna Melt Bites	Curried Chicken Salad	Orange Tequila Steak
Calories: 372 Fats: 32g Net Carbs: 6g Protein: 16g	Calories: 318 Fats: 24g Net Carbs: 3g Protein: 22g	Calories: 560 Fats: 46g Net Carbs: 6g Protein: 26g

Avocado Baked Eggs

Prep Time: 3 minutes
Cooking Time: 12 minutes
Serves: 1

Ingredients:

·   1 slice of bacon
·   ½ an avocado, not too squishy, pip removed
·   ¼ teaspoon Creole seasoning
·   1 large egg
·   1 oz. Monterey Jack cheese, shredded or sliced

Steps:

1. Preheat the oven to 400°F.
2. Fry the bacon until it is crisp.
3. Scoop out a little flesh from the cavity of the avocado to allow it to fit an egg.
4. Take a sharp knife and score the flesh of the avocado in a crisscross pattern so that you create ½ inch squares.
5. Grease a ramekin or coat it with non-stick cooking spray.
6. Place the avocado half in the ramekin.
7. Spoon some bacon grease onto the avocado, allowing it to get into the scoring. Sprinkle on the Creole seasoning.
8. Break the egg into the avocado half.
9. Place the ramekin in the oven and cook for 12 minutes. After 10 minutes, pull out and sprinkle with cheese.
10. Garnish with the bacon and serve.

Nutritional Breakdown:

372 calories, 32 grams fat, 16 grams protein, 9 grams total carbs, 3 grams dietary fiber.

Avocado Tuna Melt Bites

Prep Time: 4 minutes
Cooking Time: 7 minutes
Serves: 1

Ingredients:

- 1 can drained tuna
- ¼ cup of mayonnaise
- 1 small avocado, cubed
- ¼ cup Parmesan cheese
- ½ tablespoon garlic powder
- ¼ tablespoon onion powder
- salt and pepper to taste
- ¼ cup coconut oil for frying
- I cup almond flour

Steps:

1. Drain the tuna and place it into a large bowl.
2. Add in mayonnaise, Parmesan cheese and spices and mix well.
3. Add the avocado cubes into the mixture, without squashing them.
4. Form the mixture into balls and roll in almond flour until completely covered.
5. Heat the coconut oil in a pan and cook the tuna balls until they are crisp all over. Serve immediately.

Nutritional Breakdown:

352 calories, 36 grams fat, 25 grams protein, 14 grams total carbs, 7.5 grams dietary fiber.

Maple Flavored Pork Bake

Prep Time: 2 minutes
Cooking Time: 16 minutes
Serves: 1

Ingredients:

- 1.5 oz. 40% heavy cream, whipped
- 3 drops of vanilla flavoring
- 6 oz. ground pork, cooked
- ½ oz. macadamia nuts, crushed
- 0.4 oz. butter
- 1 oz. cheddar cheese
- pinch of calorie free sweetener

·   3 drops maple flavoring

Steps:

1.   Mix the whipped cream with the vanilla flavor and half of the sweetener.
Freeze for 15 minutes.
2.   Pre-heat the oven to 350 degrees F. In an oven safe dish, mix the pork, macadamia nuts, butter, cheese, remaining sweetener, and maple flavor. Bake for 15 minutes.
3.   Serve with the frozen whipped cream on top as ice cream.

Nutritional Breakdown:

405 calories, 37 grams fat, 17 grams protein, 6 grams total carbs, 4.1 grams dietary fiber.

Breakfast Casserole

Prep Time: 6 minutes
Cooking Time: 25 minutes
Serves: 1

Ingredients:

·   2 large eggs
·   ¼ lb. sausage
·   ½ cup of grated cheddar cheese
·   ½ cup heavy cream
·   ¼ head cauliflower
·   ¼ teaspoon dry mustard
·   ¼ teaspoon sea salt

Steps:

1.   Preheat the oven to 350°F. Grease a casserole dish or coat it with non-stick cooking spray.
2.   Place a non-stick skillet over a medium-high flame and cook the sausage until browned and crumbled.
3.   Scrape the sausage into a bowl, then stir in the chopped cauliflower, heavy cream, cheese, salt and mustard. Set aside to cool.

4.   Whisk the eggs in a separate bowl, then stir into the sausage mixture.
5.   Pour the mixture into the casserole dish. Bake for 25 minutes.
6.   Set on a wire rack to cool slightly, then serve.

Nutritional Breakdown:

311 calories, 32 grams fat, 18 grams protein, 8.6 grams total carbs, 2.8 grams dietary fiber.

Quesadilla with Creamy Mushroom Dip

Prep Time: 3 minutes
Cooking Time: 5 minutes
Serves: 1

Ingredients:

- 1/8 cup heavy duty cream
- 1 Tablespoon mayonnaise
- 1 Teaspoon olive oil
- 1 avocado
- Dollop of butter
- 2 egg whites
- 1/8 cup almond flour
- Grated cheese to garnish

Steps:

1.   Combine the cream, olive oil, avocado and mayonnaise in a mixing bowl. Mash together until smooth.
2.   In another bowl, mix the egg whites and almond flour.
3.   Melt the butter in a small non-stick fry-pan on medium heat.
4.   Pour the egg whites into the pan in a thin layer.
5.   When the egg mixture is opaque, flip and cook the other side.
6.   Remove the heat and add the cheese, sprinkling it on top.
7.   Fold in half to melt the cheese.
8.   Remove eggs from the pan and slice into wedges. Serve with avocado dip.

Nutritional Breakdown:

404 calories, 43g fat, 21g protein, 7.1g carbohydrate, 4.6g dietary fiber

Curried Chicken Salad

Prep Time: 6 minutes
Cooking Time: 30 minutes
Serves: 1

Ingredients:

- 1/4 clove garlic
- ¼ teaspoon chopped fresh ginger
- ½ teaspoon fresh lemon juice
- 1/4 teaspoon curry powder
- ¼ teaspoon Dijon mustard
- ¼ teaspoon coarse salt
- ¼ teaspoon freshly ground pepper
- ¼ cup canola oil
- 1 cup cooked and cubed chicken
- ½ cup broccoli florets, blanched for 1 minute
- ½ cup sliced celery
- ¼ cup salted cashews
- 1 cup pre-washed spinach
- Chives, to garnish

Steps:

1. To make the curry vinaigrette, chop up the garlic and ginger in a food processor. Add the lemon juice, curry, mustard and salt and pepper and blend. Pour the canola oil and process until smooth. Put this mixture in a container and cool in the fridge for an hour.
2. Combine the chicken, broccoli, celery and cashews in a large bowl. Add the curry vinaigrette and toss until well blended.
3. To serve, make a bed of the spinach on a dinner plate. Spoon the salad in the middle of the spinach. Garnish with long strands of chives.

Nutritional Breakdown:

318 calories 24g fat, 22g protein, 5g carbohydrate, 2g dietary fiber, sodium 213 mg

Tandoori Chicken

Prep Time: 5 minutes (plus refrigeration overnight)
Cooking Time: 35 minutes
Serves: 1

Ingredients:

- ¼ cup plain yogurt
- ½ tablespoon fresh lime juice
- ¼ piece of fresh ginger, peeled and minced
- ¼ garlic, minced
- ¼ teaspoon chili powder
- ¼ teaspoon coarse salt
- 1/8 teaspoon ground cumin
- 1/8 teaspoon ground turmeric
- ¼ tablespoon tandoori paste
- ¼ chicken, with all visible fat removed

Steps:

1. To make the marinade put all the ingredients excluding the chicken in a large re-sealable bag. Shake well.
2. Add the chicken and coat liberally. Refrigerate overnight.
3. Remove the chicken from the marinade and place on a grill coated with a non-stick vegetable spray over medium heat. Grill for 35 minutes. Baste a couple of times with the marinade.
4. Serve immediately.

Nutritional Breakdown:

503 calories, 30g fat, 52g protein, 4g carbohydrate, 0g dietary fiber, sodium 164 mg

Veal Picata

Prep Time: 5 minutes
Cooking Time: 8 minutes
Serves: 1

Ingredients:

- 1/4 tablespoon extra-virgin olive oil

- 1 veal scallop (6 oz.)
- 1/8 teaspoon coarse salt
- 1/8 teaspoon freshly ground pepper
- 1/8 teaspoon freshly ground coriander
- ¼ garlic clove, minced
- 1/8 cup chicken broth
- 1/8 cup fresh lemon juice
- ½ tablespoon capers, rinsed and drained
- ½ tablespoon butter
- ½ tablespoon minced fresh parsley
- thinly sliced lemon for garnish

Steps:

1.   Heat a skillet for 60 seconds. Add olive oil and swirl the pan to coat the bottom evenly. Season both sides of the veal with salt and pepper. Place the veal in the skillet and sauté for 2 minutes on each side. Remove to a plate and cover with foil.
2.   Add the garlic to the skillet and sauté for 30 seconds. Add chicken broth and cook on high for 2 minutes. Add lemon juice and capers and cook for 1 minute.
3.   Remove the skillet from the heat and add the butter. Once butter has melted add the parsley and blend.
4.   Garnish with a lemon slice to serve.

Nutritional Breakdown:

325 calories, 20g fat, 32g protein, 2g carbohydrate, 1g dietary fiber, sodium 595 mg

Pickled Salmon

Prep Time: 5 minutes (plus refrigeration overnight)
Cooking Time: 20 minutes
Serves: 1

Ingredients:

- 1/2-pound salmon steaks or skinned fillets
- 1 teaspoon salt
- 1 cup water
- 1/4 cup white vinegar
- 1/4 cup Splenda

- 1/4 bay leaf
- 1-inch piece cinnamon stick
- 1/4 slice fresh ginger crushed
- 1/4 lemon sliced
- 1/2 medium onion, thinly sliced

Steps:

1. Rub the fish with the salt and then refrigerate for one hour.
2. Combine the water, Splenda, vinegar, bay leaf, cinnamon stick, ginger and lemon in a saucepan. Bring the mixture to the boil, lower the heat and allow to simmer for 5 minutes.
3. Add the fish and simmer uncovered for another 7 minutes.
4. Place onion slices on a casserole dish and with the fish on top and cover with the hot vinegar mixture. Cover and refrigerate overnight.

Nutritional Breakdown:

370 calories, 4g fat, 23g protein, 11g carbohydrate, 4g dietary fiber, sodium 267 mg

Orange Tequila Steak

Prep Time: 5 minutes (plus overnight refrigeration)
Cooking Time: 12 minutes
Serves: 1

Ingredients:

- 1/2-pound beef steak
- 2 cloves garlic
- 1/4 cup lemon juice
- 1/4 cup lime juice
- 1 shot tequila
- 1 teaspoon chili powder
- 1/2 tablespoon Splenda
- 1 teaspoon dried oregano
- 1 1/2 tablespoons olive oil
- 1/4 teaspoon orange extract

Steps:

1.   Mix all the ingredients except the steak in a re-sealable bag and mix together. Add the steak and turn the bag to fully cover it. Place in the refrigerator to marinade overnight.
2.   Pour the marinade out into a bowl.
3.   Grill the steak for 12 minutes (6 mins per side) on medium heat.
4.   Baste at least 2 times during cooking.

Nutritional Breakdown:

560 calories, 46g fat, 26g protein, 6g carbohydrate, 1g dietary fiber, sodium 576 mg

Smoky Marinated Steak

Prep Time: 5 minutes (plus overnight refrigeration)
Cooking Time: 12 minutes
Serves: 1

Ingredients:

·   1/2-pound T-bone steak
·   1/2 tablespoon liquid smoke flavoring
·   1 teaspoon salt
·   1 clove garlic, crushed
·   1 dash pepper
·   1 teaspoon olive oil
·   1/8 teaspoon onion powder
·   1/4 cup water

Steps:

1.   Mix all the ingredients except the steak in a re-sealable bag and mix together. Add the steak and turn the bag to fully cover it. Place in the refrigerator to marinade overnight.
2.   Pour the marinade out in a bowl. Broil the steak for for six minutes on each side. Baste half way through, using the reserved marinade.
3.   Top with sautéed mushrooms.

Nutritional Breakdown:

276 calories, 20g fat, 23g protein, 1g carbohydrate, 0g dietary fiber, sodium 398 mg

Bacon Chili Burgers

Prep Time: 5 minutes (plus overnight refrigeration)
Cooking Time: 12 minutes
Serves: 1

Ingredients:

- ½ pound ground chuck steak
- 1 strip fat free bacon, cooked
- ¼ onion, diced
- 1-3 teaspoons chili garlic paste (depending on spice preference)
- Lettuce leaves

Steps:

1. Place the ground chuck, onion and chili garlic paste in a mixing bowl.
2. Crumble the bacon into the bowl. Mix together with your hands.
3. Form the mixture into a burger.
4. Cook the burgers for six minutes on an electric table-top grill.
5. Serve with lettuce leaves as burger buns.

Nutritional Breakdown:

485 calories, 38g fat,31g protein, 2g carbohydrate, 3g dietary fiber, sodium 268 mg

The Paleolithic Diet

Over the last decade, the Paleolithic diet (typically referred to as the "Paleo" diet) has become more than a diet, it has become a movement. The Paleo diet has legions of rabid adherents. The central idea of the Paleo diet is to eat foods that human beings

126

evolved over the course of millions of years to eat. In very simple terms, the aim of the Paleo diet is to eat like a caveman. That is where the Paleo diet gets its name – "paleo" is defined as "'old' or 'ancient,' especially in reference to former geologic time periods." [174] The Paleo diet is also referred to as the "Ancestral" diet, "Caveman" diet, "Primal" diet, or "Hunter-Gatherer" diet. Like many diets, there is no one central authority for all matters "Paleo". There are many debates within the Paleo community as to what specifically constitutes a true Paleo diet. There is so much back-and-forth on what exactly can earn the moniker of a true Paleo food item, the question, "Is this Paleo?", has become a sort of punchline on Paleo websites, blogs, and podcasts.

Most Paleo diet devotees would agree that it consists of meats, vegetables, and nuts and avoids grains, legumes, and dairy. There is a large emphasis within the Paleo community on eating animal meat that was raised in an evolutionarily compatible way: that means grass-fed beef and bison, wild-caught seafood, and pasture-raised poultry and pork. The well-known Paleo diet expert and author, Robb Wolf explains that a Paleo diet should include: diverse proteins including organ meats and bone broth, fruits and vegetables, and "healthy fats from nuts, seeds, avocados, olive oil, fish oil and grass-fed meat." [175]

According to another respected Paleo diet expert and author, John Durant, author of *The Paleo Manifesto: Ancient Wisdom for Lifelong Health*, an "orthodox" Paleo diet avoids "sugars (added or otherwise), vegetable oils (canola oil, soybean oil corn oil), grains (wheat, corn, oats, barley), legumes (soy, peanuts, beans), and dairy (milk, cheese)". Instead, the Paleo diet gravitates toward seafood (salmon, sardines, shellfish), meat (beef, lamb, poultry, pork), vegetables (spinach, cabbage, broccoli), roots and tubers (carrots, sweet potatoes), eggs, a little fruit (particularly berries), and a few nuts (walnuts, almonds)...fermented foods (sauerkraut, kimchi)...real animal fats and tropical oils (coconut oil, butter, beef tallow, olive oil); and...organ meats (liver, marrow, heart)." [176]

Many of the positive health claims of the Paleo diet are backed by scientific evidence. For example, a 2009 report in *The European Journal of Clinical Nutrition* found, "Even short-term consumption of a paleolithic type diet improves [blood pressure] and glucose tolerance, decreases insulin secretion, increases insulin sensitivity and improves lipid profiles without weight loss in healthy sedentary humans." [177] A study from 2015 compared diabetic patients. One group ate a Paleo diet and the other group ate a diet endorsed by the American Diabetes Association (ADA) for three weeks. By the end of the study, "Both groups had improvements in metabolic measures, but the Paleo diet group had greater benefits on glucose control and lipid profiles. Also, on the Paleo diet, the most insulin-resistant subjects had a significant improvement in insulin sensitivity ... but no such effect was seen in the most insulin-resistant subjects on the ADA diet." [178]

In 2015, *The American Journal of Clinical Nutrition* reviewed a series of randomized control trials (RCT's) comparing the Paleo diet to more traditional recommended guideline-based diets. The *Journal* found that the Paleo diet "resulted in greater short-term pooled improvements on each of the 5 components of the metabolic syndrome than did currently recommended guideline-based control diets. However, the greater pooled improvements did not reach significance for 2 of the 5 components (i.e., [high-density lipoprotein (HDL)] cholesterol and fasting blood sugar). For each metabolic syndrome component, the quality of the evidence for the pooled estimate for improvement was moderate. Furthermore, there was moderate quality evidence for greater weight loss on Paleolithic nutrition relative to the control diet." That same review went on to hypothesize that many of the benefits of the Paleo diet may spring from "the absence of processed food". It also questioned whether the exclusion of whole-grains and fermented dairy products was necessary since epidemiological data suggests that they "protect against diabetes." [179]

Middle-aged professional bodybuilder and five-time Mr. Olympia competitor Mark Dugdale, who took first place at an IFBB contest

128

as recently as June 2017 (qualifying for a sixth Olympia competition), essentially ascribes to a version of the Paleo diet as his nutritional choice. This is the way he describes his diet: "In summary, I favor a diet rich in organic, non-GMO and raw/fermented whole foods that are in-season and vibrant in color. Sugar and refined carbohydrates are the major sources of health issues ..." 180

Not all the news surrounding the Paleo diet is positive. A 2014 study, for example, published in the *International Journal of Exercise Science* found "the Paleo diet was significantly deleterious to blood lipid profiles in healthy subjects concurrently participating in a CrossFit based, high-intensity circuit training program." 181 A 2013 article in Scientific American skewered the Paleo diet and lambasted many of its principles, particularly the wholesale banning of entire food groups like dairy. The article characterized the Paleo diet as "half-baked". 182 US News and World Reports gathered a panel of health experts to rank 40 diets on several measures. The Paleo diet ranked number 32 overall and the highest ordering it received was a measly number 29 on the list of "Easiest Diets to Follow". On the list of "Best Heart-Healthy Diets", it earned a low 35th place ranking out of 40. 183

The Mediterranean Diet

Another option to consider is the Mediterranean diet. The same US News and World Report survey that ranked the Paleo diet number 32 overall, pegged the Mediterranean diet as the best overall diet out of the 40 diets evaluated. It was also ranked number one in several sub-categories like "Best Diets for Healthy Eating", "Easiest Diets to Follow", and "Best Plant-Based Diets". 184

There really is not one specific diet that can be officially labeled as "The Mediterranean Diet". However, the Mediterranean diet is described in an article from *The American Journal of Clinical Nutrition* as a diet "characterized by abundant plant foods (fruit, vegetables, breads, other forms of cereals, potatoes, beans, nuts, and seeds), fresh fruit as the typical daily dessert, olive oil as the principal source of fat, dairy products (principally cheese and yogurt), and fish and poultry consumed in low to moderate amounts, zero to four eggs consumed weekly, red meat consumed in low amounts, and wine consumed in low to moderate amounts, normally with meals. This diet is low in saturated fat (< or = 7-8% of energy), with total fat ranging from < 25% to > 35% of energy throughout the region." [185]

The focus on wholesome, natural and unprocessed foods along with a moderate intake of healthy fats, specifically olive oil, is a distinguishing feature of the Mediterranean diet. The use of olive oil in the diet, replacing butter, margarine and other types of less healthy fats, helps to increase the functioning of HDL, the good cholesterol in the body.

Like other healthy diet options, the Mediterranean diet includes lean proteins like fish, poultry and limited red meat. The bulk of the meal is made up of plant-based food choices such as fruits, vegetables and whole grains. Legumes and nuts are also included in this diet.

Typically, dairy and red meat are limited. Salt is also limited, but natural herbs and spices are encouraged. Many organizations, including the American Heart Association as well as the American Diabetes Association, support this diet.

The science surrounding the Mediterranean diet is encouraging. A 2004 study in the *Journal of the American Medical Association* concluded "Among individuals aged 70 to 90 years, adherence to a Mediterranean diet and healthful lifestyle is associated with a more than 50% lower rate of all-causes and cause-specific mortality." [186] Likewise, a 2013 study from *The New England Journal of Medicine* discovered that, "Among persons at high cardiovascular risk, a Mediterranean diet supplemented with extra-virgin olive oil or nuts reduced the incidence of major cardiovascular events." [187] The journal *Annals of Neurology* surveyed 2,258 people over the course of four years and determined "that higher adherence to the [Mediterranean diet] is associated with a reduction in risk for [Alzheimer's disease]." [188] In a separate evaluation of the Mediterranean diet, investigators compared the impact of the moderate-fat Mediterranean diet to a standard low-fat diet on 101 overweight men and women for 18 months. At the conclusion of the investigation, the subjects on the Mediterranean had lost weight and inches from their waist. However, the low-fat diet group gained weight and increased their waist size. [189]

The Big Picture

The big idea with nutrition is to stop "dieting" and instead create a way of eating that becomes a lifestyle. The goal is to develop a realistic, healthy approach to adding the macronutrients and micronutrients you need for your workout, life and your goals.

Changing your thinking from dieting, which means a stop and a start point, to making a lifestyle change is one of the most effective ways to make a real switch in your food intake. Becoming conscious of why you are eating specific foods and not just mindlessly grazing throughout the day can mark a major turning point for most people, particularly those who are dealing with metabolisms that may be naturally slowing and muscle loss that is making fat burning less efficient.

Adding exercise and weight lifting will boost muscle growth and fat burning, but you need to give it the right fuel. Unless you are competitively lifting, extreme diets and high levels of protein intake is not helpful to your overall goals and may cause additional challenges to reaching your goals.

Perhaps Danny Lennon, the respected host of Sigma Nutrition Radio, sums it up best in his insightful article "The Ridiculously Simple Guide to Sustainable Fat Loss," when he says:

"Eat mostly natural, whole foods, hit a suitable intake of calories and protein, sleep 7-9 hours a night, do some form of exercise and don't stress over unimportant things. Do that and repeat each day." [190]

Supplements

If there seems to be a lot of confusion and conflicting information about diet and nutrition in weight loss and muscle gain, there is even more hype and misinformation about supplements. The supplement industry sold more than 36 billion dollars' worth of vitamins and nutritional supplements in the US in 2017 and that number continues to grow every year. [191] Nearly every fitness and bodybuilding publication and web site is hawking some sort of supplement or receiving some kind of affiliate marketing income from advertising supplements. It is in the interest of supplement companies to wow you with extraordinary claims of increased muscle growth, unlimited energy, or nearly instant fat-melting. If only the frothy claims matched the reality.

But, the truth is there is no magic elixir or combination of compounds that can be taken, shaken, injected or consumed in any fashion that will trigger incredible fat loss and muscle growth on their own. The single best supplement has been, is, and for the foreseeable future, will remain to be your own discipline regarding educating yourself, eating the right foods, working hard and smart in the gym, getting quality sleep, and maintaining a winning attitude. With that in mind, there are some supplements that have been proven to provide some degree of an edge in our quests to get ripped.

Before we begin our discussion of those supplements, though, caution must be taken. Some supplements, in fact, are dangerous and potentially life-threatening. Dietary supplements in the US are not regulated by the US Food and Drug Administration (FDA). There is no assurance of safety. In 2014, supplements caused 20% of all drug-induced liver injuries. Two supplements in particular pose "unique threats to the liver: anabolic steroids, which are sometimes illegally added to bodybuilding supplements; and green tea extract, which is found in many weight-loss supplements." [192] A case study from the *Canadian Journal of Gastroenterology*, for example, details the story of a "previously healthy 28-year old female bodybuilder with no risk factors for liver disease [who] presented to her local emergency room centre with fatigue, malaise, inability to exercise, and new-onset jaundice. Her symptoms worsened over a span of one week before hospitalization." She had been taking a fat-burner containing green tea extract, usnic acid, and guggul tree extract (there are still supplements available for sale containing these ingredients). She eventually lapsed into a semi-coma and required a breathing tube. After an emergency liver transplant, she regained consciousness and was eventually discharged from the hospital. [193]

Supplements also do not necessarily list all ingredients on the label. The FDA reports that some supplements "contain a wide variety of undeclared active pharmaceutical ingredients." So, even if you know that you need to avoid ingredients like green tea extract, usnic acid, and guggul tree extract, your supplement may include those same or other harmful ingredients. For example, a police sergeant in Baltimore lost his job because he took a weight-loss supplement that he did not realize contained an amphetamine banned by his department as an unlisted ingredient. [194]

It is also important to remember that using any type of supplement means following the instructions. If you are "stacking" your supplements – taking multiple supplements together – be aware that the combinative effects of certain supplements may produce undesirable results. Also, remember that the dose-relationship of many supplements follows the pattern of a "hormetic" inverted U-shaped curve. In other words, there is an optimum dose. Exceeding that dose does not yield additional benefits and can cause harm.

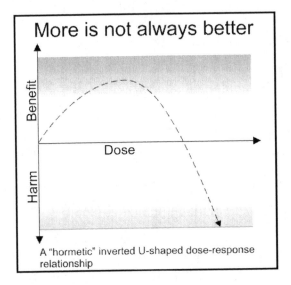

A "hormetic" inverted U-shaped dose-response relationship

There are, however, some supplements that can be beneficial to achieving weight loss and muscle growth goals. These are not stand-alone components and need to be integrated with a healthy diet and exercise to see results. Think of supplements as the icing on the cake of your diet, exercise, sleep, and stress-reduction lifestyle – they are worthless without the cake.

Do your research and learn about any possible risks or complications that may occur with a specific supplement based on your own health profile. My personal first place to turn to research a supplement is Examine.com. ConsumerLab.com is also a very helpful site that provides safety and efficacy analyses of many different nutritional supplements. If you have any doubts or any kind of medical condition, always consult with a doctor first.

There are seemingly innumerable supplements available with all kinds of claims about their beneficial effects. We will look at a few of the most well-studied supplements with solid scientific evidence behind their reported benefits. It would require at least several hundred pages to adequately address each supplement available on the market. None of this is meant to be a recommendation to consume these supplements and, as mentioned above, always review the supplement, the manufacturer and consider any risks or health issues before starting use.

Creatine

Creatine is a naturally occurring substance that is made in the liver and kidneys from the amino acids glycine, arginine, and methionine. [195] In foods, it can be found in low amounts in nuts, meat, dairy and fish.

In a previous section of this book, we discussed the ATP-PC energy delivery system. To recap, the ATP-PC system fuels the body's energy requirements during the first 10-15 seconds of activity, especially intense activity. The ATP-PC system is the body's quickest way to deliver energy. It also produces the most power output compared to the body's three other energy delivery systems, or "gears".

The ATP-PC system relies on two biochemical components to function: adenosine triphosphate (ATP) and phosphocreatine (PC) stored in the muscle fibrils, specifically the myosin portion of the sarcomere. ATP is the body's energy currency. As it is brought out of storage within the muscle fibril to be consumed by the muscle for use as energy, it is stripped of one of its phosphates (Pi) to become adenosine diphosphate (ADP). Meanwhile, PC is broken down into creatine and Pi. "The energy released in the breakdown of PC allows ADP and Pi to rejoin forming more ATP.

This newly formed ATP can now be broken down to release energy to fuel activity." [196] By this process, creatine effectively recycles the ATP stored in the muscles and acts a as a sort of human energy force multiplier for the ATP-PC cycle. It stands to reason, then, that the more creatine that is available in muscle tissue to recycle ATP, the more energy that will be produced during the ATP-PC cycle.

Creatine supplementation increases the concentration of total creatine levels in muscle tissue. A 1994 review article from the journal *Sports Medicine* cited four different studies showing creatine supplementation over periods varying from five days to thirty days increased creatine levels by 8% to almost 20% in muscle tissue versus control subjects. [197] As explained above, by increasing the amount of creatine stored in the muscle tissue, supplementation increases the amount of PC available to donate a phosphate (Pi) to ADP to convert it back into ATP. This provides additional fuel for the ATP-PC process.

In 2007, the *Journal of the International Society of Sports Nutrition* released a position stand on creatine supplementation and exercise. In that position stand, the Society made several points regarding creatine supplementation. Some of those points were:

> 1. Creatine monohydrate is the most effective ergogenic nutritional supplement currently available to athletes in terms of increasing high-intensity exercise capacity and lean body mass during training.
> 2. Creatine monohydrate supplementation is not only safe, but possibly beneficial in regard to preventing injury and/or management of select medical conditions when taken within recommended guidelines.
> 3. There is no scientific evidence that the short- or long-term use of creatine monohydrate has any detrimental effects on otherwise healthy individuals.
> ...

5. At present, creatine monohydrate is the most extensively studied and clinically effective form of creatine for use in nutritional supplements in terms of muscle uptake and ability to increase high-intensity exercise capacity.

6. The addition of carbohydrate or carbohydrate and protein to a creatine supplement appears to increase muscular retention of creatine, although the effect on performance measures may not be greater than using creatine monohydrate alone.

7. The quickest method of increasing muscle creatine stores appears to be to consume ~0.3 grams/kg/day of creatine monohydrate for at least 3 days followed by 3–5 g/d thereafter to maintain elevated stores. Ingesting smaller amounts of creatine monohydrate (e.g., 2–3 g/d) will increase muscle creatine stores over a 3–4 week period, however, the performance effects of this method of supplementation are less supported. [198]

Creatine has been studied for nearly 200 years. It was originally discovered in 1832 by Michel Chevreul, a French scientist. [199] Since that time, the pace of investigation into the function of creatine has continued to accelerate. A search on Google Scholar for "creatine supplementation" reveals approximately 52,300 results.

Several studies have specifically examined the impact of creatine supplementation on older people. A 1998 study from the *Journal of Applied Physiology* determined that older individuals (58 ± 4 years old) have a lower resting muscle creatine concentration compared to younger individuals (30 ± 5 years old) and that older people also have a lower ability to resynthesize PC after exercise. Creatine supplementation, however, eliminated the difference in resting creatine concentration and increased the level of PC resynthesis after exercise. Creatine supplementation increased the mean time to exhaustion in both the young and old groups by 30%. The study concluded, "The results of this study indicated that middle-aged persons had greater improvements in muscle [PC] availability, [PC] hydrolysis during exercise, and initial [PC] resynthesis rate after creatine supplementation, compared with younger persons, and that creatine supplementation improved muscle endurance capacity in both groups combined." [200]

Furthermore, a 2016 study out of Iran found that creatine supplementation reduced the rate of cell death ("apoptosis") as a result of acute exercise in middle-aged men. [201] And a 2000 study from the journal *Medicine and Science in Sports and Exercise* evaluated 23 trained young men over the course of six weeks of creatine supplementation. The supplemented group showed strength gains 11.8% greater than the control group. Also, the supplemented group showed marked increases in fat-free mass – for example, "upper arm muscle area increased by 11% for [the creatine group] with no change for Placebo. Creatine appear[ed] to directly stimulate increases in the size of the existing musculature." [202] Finally, a 2016 research review from *Sports Nutrition and Therapy* reported, "Supplementation with [creatine] has been advocated to improve both short-term and intermittent high intensity exercise, with some supporting literature for both mid and long-term bouts. Currently, no scientific evidence exists showing any unfavorable effects, even when supplementation is prolonged, providing correct protocols are followed and the participant is otherwise healthy." [203]

Interestingly, a 2017 study examined the impact of "stacking" caffeine with creatine. It concluded, "The findings indicate that the consumption of caffeine at 6 mg·kg^{-1} in association with 3 g of creatine for 7 days generated a significant improvement in performance, increased the production of torque, and improved the EMG muscle activity. Thus, it is more than reasonable to conclude that caffeine potentiates the effects of creatine during a physical exercise." [204] Note that the dosing recommended by the study is six milligrams per tenth of a kilogram. Therefore, a 180-pound man would dose with just under 50 milligrams of caffeine. Eight fluid ounces of coffee has almost twice as much caffeine as that dose.

Not only can creatine improve exercise performance, strength, and muscle size, but research is beginning to show that it has a wide range of other positive effects on the body. For example, a peer-reviewed 2014 study from *F1000 Research* explained, "In relation to the brain, creatine has been shown to have antioxidant properties, reduce mental fatigue, protect the brain from neurotoxicity, and improve facets/components of neurological disorders like depression and bipolar disorder. The combination of these benefits has made creatine a leading candidate in the fight against age-related diseases, such as Parkinson's disease, Huntington's disease, amyotrophic lateral sclerosis, long-term memory impairments associated with the progression of Alzheimer's disease, and stroke." [205] A 2003 study appearing in *Proceedings of The Royal Society B: Biological Sciences* found, "Creatine supplementation had a significant positive effect ... on both working memory (backward digit span) and intelligence (Raven's Advanced Progressive Matrices), both tasks that require speed of processing. These findings underline a dynamic and significant role of brain energy capacity in influencing brain performance ... This study showed that increasing creatine intake by oral supplementation resulted in improved brain function, similar to effects shown previously in muscle and heart." [206]

Creatine has more science behind it than virtually any other nutritional supplement and has been proven to provide numerous benefits. However, that does not mean it is safe for you especially if you have an existing condition particularly in your liver or kidneys. As always, know your body and exercise caution.

Beta-Alanine (β-Alanine)

Another supplement that may be beneficial is beta-alanine. Like creatine, beta-alanine has been the subject of hundreds of scientific studies. Its effects have been highly scrutinized. According to Examine.com, "Beta-alanine has been shown to enhance muscular endurance. Many people report being able to perform one or two additional reps in the gym when training in sets of 8–15 repetitions. Beta-alanine supplementation can also improve moderate- to high-intensity cardiovascular exercise performance, like rowing or sprinting." [207]

Recall from our discussion of the body's four different energy delivery systems that part of the anaerobic system is the "anaerobic glycolysis system" or "lactic acid system." The lactic acid system becomes the predominant source of energy for the body after the ATP-PC system exhausts itself. It begins to kick in at around ten seconds of sustained intense activity and continues to supply energy to the body until about 45 seconds of maximum effort activity. One of the byproducts of anaerobic glycolysis is lactic acid (the burning feeling – also called "acidosis" - in your muscles during intense exercise). As the anaerobic glycolysis system continues to supply energy to the body, lactate builds up in the muscle until "we reach a point where we cannot remove enough lactate from our muscles to control the acidosis …" At that point, the build up of lactate in the muscle reaches a point where "we are unable to sustain the intensity of exercise and have to either cease exercise or reduce the intensity." [208]

It is during this process of anaerobic glycolysis that beta-alanine becomes a performance enhancer. How?

Beta-alanine is used in the body to manufacture carnosine. A 2010 report published in *Medicine and Science in Sports and Exercise* explains, "Intramuscular acidosis has been attributed to be one of the main causes of fatigue during intense exercise. Carnosine has been shown to play a significant role in muscle pH regulation. Carnosine is synthesized in skeletal muscle from the amino acids L-histidine and β-alanine. The rate-limiting factor of carnosine synthesis is β-alanine availability. Supplementation with β-alanine has been shown to increase muscle carnosine content and therefore total muscle buffer capacity, with the potential to elicit improvements in physical performance during high-intensity exercise." [209]

Carnosine, by buffering decreasing pH levels, delays the point at which lactic acid builds up beyond a critical level. As a result, performance is enhanced: we can get an extra couple of repetitions on a set or endure for a few more seconds of HIIT before we reach the point of exhaustion. A 2006 study from the *Journal of Strength and Conditioning Research* found that 28 days of beta-alanine supplementation (at 3.2 grams per day) resulted in a "significant" 14.5% increase in neuromuscular fatigue threshold. [210]

A 2011 study, also from the *Journal of Strength and Conditioning Research*, determined that beta-alanine "appears to have the ability to augment performance and stimulate lean mass accrual in a short amount of time (8 weeks) in previously trained athletes." The athletes in that study who supplemented with four grams per day of beta-alanine, on average, increased athletic performance and gained more lean body mass than the placebo group. [211]

A 2015 study out of Australia published in the *European Journal of Sport Science* assessing the impact of beta-alanine supplementation on cyclists discovered "β- alanine supplementation significantly extended supramaximal cycling [time to exhaustion] and may have provided a worthwhile improvement to 4-km [time trial] performance." [212]

A helpful way to think of beta-alanine supplementation may be to think of it as a way to augment your body's anaerobic glycolysis system in a very similar fashion to the way creatine magnifies the ability of your body's ATP-PC system to deliver energy to your body.

Branched Chain Amino Acids

Branched chain amino acids, more commonly known as BCAAs, include valine, isoleucine and leucine. All three are essential amino acids (EAA's) and share a similar structure. What also distinguishes BCAAs from other amino acids is that they are metabolized primarily in muscle, as opposed to the liver, where the body processes other amino acids. [213] Like creatine and beta-alanine, they are one of the more heavily researched supplements available on the market.

One of the primary avenues by which BCAAs can aid muscular hypertrophy is by ingesting them during a workout. Gym bro's and bodybuilders call this an "intra" or intra-workout supplement. BCAAs are useful during a workout because "during exercise, muscle protein synthesis decreases together with a net increase in protein degradation and stimulation of BCAA oxidation." [214] That sets the stage for a catabolic (muscle-degrading) state. Ingesting BCAAs during a workout can combat the catabolic effects of a workout: "they can directly stimulate the pathways of protein synthesis. In fact, supplementing with BCAAs during exercise can help keep the muscle in a positive state of muscle protein balance, just like supplementing with a [whey protein hydrolysate]. The most important BCAA when it comes to stimulating muscle building is leucine, which acts directly to activate several key pathways of muscle building. Evidence suggests that the ratio of BCAA is important for maximizing results. A ratio of 2:1:1 of leucine to isoleucine and valine is often used to stimulate protein synthesis efficiently. Many BCAA powders come in this ratio." [215]

In 1994, the *American Journal of Physiology, Endocrinology, and Metabolism* published a study confirming that BCAA supplementation resulted in higher levels of BCAAs in the bloodstream during exercise which resulted "in a suppression of endogenous muscle protein breakdown during exercise." [216]

A 2006 study from *The Journal of Nutrition* found BCAAs, "particularly leucine, have anabolic effects on protein metabolism by increasing the rate of protein synthesis and decreasing the rate of protein degradation in resting human muscle. Also, during recovery from endurance exercise, BCAAs were found to have anabolic effects in human muscle." [217] In simple terms, muscular hypertrophy occurs when muscle protein synthesis minus muscle protein degradation is greater than zero. So, the finding that BCAAs increase protein synthesis and decrease protein degradation is very good news for muscular hypertrophy and getting ripped. And, the additional finding that BCAAs have an anabolic (muscle-building) effect on muscle during recovery from endurance exercise is doubly good news.

In 2010, the *Journal of Strength and Conditioning Research* reported, "short-term amino acid supplementation, which is high in BCAA, may produce a net anabolic hormonal profile while attenuating training-induced increases in muscle tissue damage. Athletes' nutrient intake, which periodically increases amino acid intake to reflect the increased need for recovery during periods of overreaching, may increase subsequent competitive performance while decreasing the risk of injury or illness." [218]

A second 2006 study from *The Journal of Nutrition* demonstrated "that BCAA supplementation prior to squat exercise decreased [delayed-onset muscle soreness] and muscle fatigue occurring for a few days after exercise" suggesting that BCAAs are useful for recovery after exercise. [219] A separate study published in 2006 in the *International Journal of Sport Nutrition and Exercise Metabolism* logged nearly the same finding: "amino acid supplementation attenuates [delayed-onset muscle soreness] and muscle damage when ingested in recovery days." [220]

BCAAs are one of the basic supplements that many gym-goers and bodybuilders employ to maximize their gains. You may find that they are helpful for you as well.

Summary on Supplements

Like diet, it is important to take a big picture look at supplementation as it relates to your food intake and your fitness goals. Always do your research on any supplements, including researching the manufacturer, and make choices that are based on your own health and understanding of the benefits and possible risks associated with any supplement.

It is also essential to look closely at the recommendations for use. This includes both the amount of the supplement as well as the timing of the intake of the supplement. Not all supplements should be taken pre-workout and not all are effective when taken post-workout.

4. Motivation for Lifestyle Changes

Anti-Aging

Aging is a subject that provokes a host of emotions. Many people have a stoic attitude toward it: since it is inevitable, the only logical response is to accept it and embrace it. Other people simply do not like to think about it: they box it away in their minds and ignore it. And still others celebrate it, extolling aging as a person's "golden years".

Make no mistake about it, however. Physical aging is not pretty. It is ugly. Dr Bill Andrews, one of the preeminent anti-aging scientists in the world, describes physical aging this way:

> Every single system in your body progressively fails. Your skin wrinkles; your hair whitens and falls out. Your internal organs shrink and stop functioning correctly. Your bones become porous. Your eyesight and hearing start to shut down. You energy level plummets. Your muscles atrophy. Even your mind – your memories, your personality, the very core of your identity – falls into decline. You slowly waste away, and you die. There's no sugar-coating it; aging is horrible. We often don't think about the level of suffering that aging brings because we don't see it. The people who are truly suffering are hidden away from the public view in hospices, assisted living homes, and nursing care facilities. I personally have a lot of experience visiting people in these places. They are miserable. [221]

Many people respond to this picture of aging fatalistically by asking rhetorical questions like, "Who wants to live to be 100 years old?", or making statements like, "I don't want to live past 75."

What most people do not seem to take into consideration in their orientation toward aging is the distinction between "lifespan" and "healthspan". Lifespan is exactly what it sounds like – the time between birth and death. Healthspan, though, is "the period of one's life during which one is generally healthy and free from serious disease." [222] There can be a substantial difference between lifespan and healthspan for human beings. My father, for example, died at age 79. That was his lifespan. However, for approximately the last fifteen years of his life, he suffered from Parkinson's disease. In that sense, then, we might say his healthspan was only 64 years.

The focus of Dr Andrews' research for the last 25 years has been concentrated on the role of telomeres in aging. Most people I have talked to have not heard of a "telomere" and very few people have any idea what a telomere is.

The 2009 Nobel Prize in Physiology or Medicine was awarded to three researchers, Elizabeth Blackburn, Carol Greider, and Jack Szoztak, for their research on telomeres and an enzyme called "telomerase". From the 2009 Nobel Prize citation:

> The long, thread-like DNA molecules that carry our genes are packed into chromosomes, the telomeres being the caps on their ends. Elizabeth Blackburn and Jack Szostak discovered that a unique DNA sequence in the telomeres protects the chromosomes from degradation. Carol Greider and Elizabeth Blackburn identified telomerase, the enzyme that makes telomere DNA. These discoveries explained how the ends of the chromosomes are protected by the telomeres and that they are built by telomerase.
>
> If the telomeres are shortened, cells age. Conversely, if telomerase activity is high, telomere length is maintained, and cellular senescence is delayed. This is the case in

cancer cells, which can be considered to have eternal life. Certain inherited diseases, in contrast, are characterized by a defective telomerase, resulting in damaged cells.

As we age, our telomeres shorten. In general, a young child's telomeres are longer than a middle-aged adult's telomeres which are, in turn, generally longer than an elderly person's telomeres. Science has established that there is a direct relationship between telomere length and an individual's biological age (as opposed to chronological age). Young children, for example, who suffer from progeria – "a rare congenital abnormality characterized by premature and rapid aging, the affected individual appearing in childhood as an aged person and having a shortened lifespan" [223] - "have much shorter telomeres" than children without progeria. [224] In effect, children with progeria are biologically much older than their peers.

Once a telomere shrinks to a critically short length termed "senescence", further cell replication is prevented "allowing DNA damage to occur unrepaired.". [225] This is when bad things in terms of aging start to occur. We want to delay the point in time at which our telomeres arrive at senescence as long as possible.

To give you an idea of the difference longer telomeres make, consider the story of a laboratory experiment using telomerase to lengthen human telomeres:

> ... scientists inserted the telomerase gene into human skin cells that already had very short telomeres. These cells were then grown into skin on the back of mice. As you might expect, the skin from cells that hadn't received the telomerase gene looked like old skin. It was wrinkled, it blistered easily, and it had gene expression patterns indicative of old skin. The skin grown from cells that had received the telomerase gene, in contrast, looked young. It acted like young skin, and its gene expression patterns were almost identical to the gene expression patterns of

young skin. For the first time, scientists had demonstrably reversed aging in human cells. [226]

What does all of this have to do with getting ripped past age 45? Good question. The answer is working out, especially after age 40, has been proven to be associated with longer telomeres as we age. Longer telomeres equals younger gene expression. Younger gene expression means more testosterone, less muscle wasting, better cellular repair, quicker recovery, etc, etc.

A study conducted in 2015 and published in *PLoS One* investigated the relationship between physical activity and sports participation among a cohort of 815 people all over the age of 61. The researchers queried the participants with a survey designed to assess their history of physical and sports activity. The scientists determined that telomere lengths were longest for subjects who participated in intensive activity sports and who had been physically active since at least 42 years of age. Interestingly, members of the study cohort who had participated in sports only between the ages of 20 and 30 showed no benefit in terms of telomere length. Their telomeres were the same length as compared to those who had engaged in "no sports at all ... Physical activity is clearly associated with longer [telomere length]." The researchers continued, "Our data suggest that regular physical activity for at least 10 years is necessary to achieve a sustained effect on [telomere length]. [227] A separate study in 2015 examined whether having been an elite-class athlete in early life might have an impact on telomere length in later life. The results of this study matched with the above study and found no relationship between having participated in vigorous athletic activity earlier in life and telomere length later. [228] In terms of aging, it seems, there is no resting on your laurels.

Other researchers, including Nobel Prize laureate Elizabeth Blackburn, examined the relationship between stress, exercise, and aging. They determined that, as expected, stress results in shorter telomeres. However, what is very compelling is that they discovered that exercise mitigates and, depending on the type and amount of exercise, eliminates the telomere-shortening impact of stress. The researchers ascertained that for "those who exercised less than the recommended amount, a one unit increase in the perceived stress scale ... was related to a 15-fold increase in the odds of having short telomeres." Furthermore, the scientists were able to determine that, "At values of exercise below 42 minutes across the three days, perceived stress was significantly related to the odds of having short [telomere length]. On the other hand, at values higher than 42 minutes, perceived stress was unrelated to [telomere length] ... Thus, at least 14 minutes a day of vigorous exercise appears to be a critical amount for protection from the effects of stress." [229] Note that the researchers were using US Centers for Disease Control (CDC) definitions of activity intensity. According to the CDC, "vigorous" activity is defined as burning more than seven calories per minutes. Activities like walking faster than five miles per hour, jogging or running, circuit weight training, boxing, wrestling, and CrossFit (vigorous calisthenics and weight-training) would all qualify as vigorous activity. [230]

In a 2008 study published in the *Archives of Internal Medicine*, researchers discovered that the more inactive a person is as they age, the shorter their telomeres are, and the more risk they will be at risk for age-related diseases. The study looked at body mass index (BMI), as well as other habits such as smoking in relation to physical activity. What was found is no surprise: with an increase in BMI, increased inactivity, and a sedentary lifestyle, there was a negative effect on telomere length, which means an acceleration of aging. [231]

Finally, a study published in 2017 in *Medicine and Science in Sports and Exercise* looked into the association between different types of physical activity and telomere length. "On average, an increase of [one hour per week] of vigorous [leisure time physical activity] was associated with" longer telomeres. Moreover, exceeding the recommended level of physical activity of 300 minutes per week was linked with longer telomeres while those not meeting the physical activity levels (150-300 minutes per week) or not exceeding the levels showed no difference in telomere length. [232] In other words, unless you engaged in at least 300 minutes per week of vigorous activity, there was no benefit to your telomeres.

What this research indicates is that vigorous physical activity, especially in your 40's and beyond is vitally important to how long you will live and your ability to avoid age-related diseases. This is a powerful motivator for anyone, but particularly for Dads who want to be able not just to be present at special events in their kids' lives, but to have the ability to enjoy them and be physically able to participate and have fun.

Motivation Evolution

Motivation is where this book started, and where it will end. Without a deep, personal, and meaningful reason, it is highly unlikely that you will persist for the long haul that is required to reshape your body. This is real work. This is a real challenge. You will battle against your own laziness and excuses. There will be days you will not want to go to the gym. There will be days you will not want to stick to the diet. It is on those days that the battle is won or lost. Each time you shrink back from the challenge, you make it easier to falter the next time.

Ultimately, this is not about aesthetics. This is truly a fight for your life. Look around you. It is undeniable that most men past the age of 45 have given up – at least on maintaining their bodies. And if their bodies are any reflection at all of other areas of their lives, then Henry David Thoreau had it right when he famously said, "The mass of men lead lives of quiet desperation."

According to the CDC, the average American man over the age of 20 is 5 feet, 9 inches tall, weighs 196 pounds, and has a waist size of 40 inches. [233] Gentlemen, with those numbers, that average American guy is virtually guaranteed to develop some sort of disease(s) and/or disorder(s) of lifestyle: type II diabetes, sarcopenia, heart disease, stroke, rheumatoid arthritis, cancer, hypertension, Alzheimer's, Parkinson's, etc. Yes, our genetic profile makes some of us more at risk for certain diseases and disorders than average. However, "less than 5% of the typically Western diseases are primarily attributable to genetic factors". [234] You absolutely can mitigate that risk through your lifestyle choices.

The field of "epigenetics" is able to explain how it is possible to have the genetic code that predisposes you to a particular disease but never actually manifest it. Epigenetics studies how genes express themselves. Think about it, when you are born, your genetic code is already established. However, most toddlers do not have gray hair. Most little boys are not bald. Fast-forward sixty years and many of those toddlers will have gray hair and some of those little boys will be bald. Yet the little children and the older versions of themselves have the exact same genetic code both when they are very young and when they are older. Why do they look so different? Epigenetics explains why: their genes are expressing differently sixty years later. For example, the little toddler had the gene that allowed for the development of gray hair, but that gene did not express itself until decades later. Likewise, you may have the gene(s) for Alzheimer's disease but it does not have to express itself.

Another way to think about epigenetics is to think of your genetic code as a blueprint for a beautiful mansion. The quality of the materials you decide to build the mansion with and the skill of the laborers you hire to construct the mansion will have a major impact on how long and how well the mansion holds up over time. If the blueprint calls for fine Italian marble floors and stainless-steel rebar in the concrete foundation but you elect to provide the workers with linoleum flooring and decide to skip paying for the stainless-steel rebar and go with a cut-rate rebar instead, how long do you think it will be before the mansion begins to show its age and fall apart? One person may think their blueprint for their mansion is not as beautiful as another person's blueprint for their mansion. However, if the first person takes care to use quality materials and highly-skilled workers and the second person employs a low-ball, cut-rate, budget strategy to build their mansion, which mansion is more likely to crumble and decline over the years?

You have a choice in the way you treat your body and the choice is entirely yours. You must decide if it is worth it to you to put in the work. What do you want for yourself? In the novel *Fight Club* by Chuck Palahniuk, there is a classic line which is entirely apropos to this conversation: "If you don't know what you want … you end up with a lot you don't." [235] What are your goals? What are your standards? What are you willing to accept for yourself? Are you willing to go down without a fight? Are you willing to put in the time, effort, and sacrifice for a bright, healthy, and vital future for yourself?

What are the costs for you if you do not begin to take action to get fit? Think of some of them: struggling with diseases and disorders that are virtually guaranteed to arise from a sedentary lifestyle, feeling sluggish and out of breath from minimal exertion, feeling tired and out of energy, looking old and unattractive. Those are just a few of the costs. There are more. Yes, it will cost you time and energy to get up and get to the gym. But it will also cost you dearly if you do not do so.

Do you think you do not have the time to work out? A study from 2012 calculated that just over ten minutes of walking per day can add nearly two years to your life. An hour per day can add 4.5 years. Up the intensity of your physical activity and you can add more than seven years to your lifespan. [236] Do you think you might want that time?

Do you have kids? What kind of example are you setting for them if you have acquiesced to middle age, letting your body go amidst the pressures of career and family? Take the example of Otis "Hoop" Hooper: he was seventeen years into his career as a US Air Force pilot and had let himself slide under the pressure of his job and home life. He explains, "I was so busy that I'd eat whatever was convenient – usually fast food."

As a father of four boys, Hoop wanted his sons to know the value of "working hard, playing hard, and eating smart." One day, in a talk with his boys intended to impart some of those values on them, Hoop's son Izaac poked his finger into Hoop's corpulent paunch.

"What about you?", Izaac asked Hoop. "Hooper came to the same realization that a lot of fathers eventually reach: He was being watched. All the time ... What his kids saw was a tired, out-of-shape guy who wasn't keeping up the way he used to." [237]

For Hoop, that lit a fire inside of him and provided the motivation he needed to completely reconstruct himself in one of the most amazing body transformation stories of all time. Eighteen months after that conversation with his sons, Hoop had entirely shed his dad bod losing fifty pounds of fat and gaining twenty-five pounds of muscle. Even more amazingly, during those same eighteen months, Hoop became an IFBB professional athlete, and qualified for and competed in the 2016 Mr Olympia contest in the physique division.

To give you some perspective on the magnitude of Hoop's accomplishments, to become an IFBB professional athlete, "a bodybuilder must earn an IFBB Pro card. In order to get the card, a bodybuilder has to win a regional contest weight class. This will earn them an invite into a national championship. Depending on the federation, if you win overall champion at the contest you will earn an IFBB Pro card." [238] None of those hurdles are easy to clear.

Qualifying for the Mr Olympia contest – the pinnacle of bodybuilding – is even more difficult than becoming an IFBB professional. Some professional bodybuilders work their entire careers – years – without ever making the cut for the Olympia. Hoop did it in an absolutely astounding eighteen months. To qualify for the Olympia competition, a competitor must fit into one of the following criteria:

> 1. The top 6 finalists from the previous year's Mr. Olympia.
> 2. The top 5 finalists from the same year's Arnold Schwarzenegger Classic and Night of the Champions.
> 3. The top 3 finalists from any Grand Prix or other professional bodybuilding competition held subsequent to the previous year's Mr. Olympia.
> 4. The overall winner from the same year's Masters Olympia.
> 5. Any former Mr. Olympia winner has a lifetime eligibility.
> 6. The Organizer may, with the approval of the Pro Committee, extend one "special invitation" to an athlete who has not qualified in accordance with the above criteria. [239]

Hoop has gone on to compete on the television show, *American Ninja Warrior*, was named one of *Men's Health* magazine's Ultimate Men's Health Guy finalists for 2016, completed an Ironman triathlon, and has had roles in major motion pictures. The genesis for all of that was the desire to be a better role model for his four sons. Can you find a similar motivation?

You're fantastic for reading my book! I'd like to ask you for a favor

If you enjoyed *Ripped Dad: Fit After 45*, then would you be kind enough to leave a review for it on Amazon? It'd be greatly appreciated! I check all my reviews and love to hear feedback. It brings me great joy to hear how everyone has benefited from this book. Just go to your account on Amazon and leave a review for *Ripped Dad: Fit After 45*. Thank you and good luck

FREE KETOGENIC COOKBOOK!

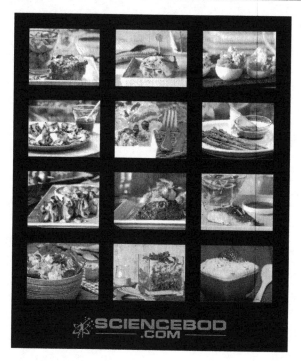

Please visit ScienceBod.com to sign up for our mailing list to receive your free fat-melting ketogenic cookbook loaded with delicious fat-burning recipes and for a chance to receive free review copies of our upcoming books.

Endnotes

[1] Vermeulen A, Goemaere S, Kaufman JM. "Testosterone, body composition and aging." *Journal of Endocrinological Investigation*: Volume 22(5 Suppl), 01 Jan 1999. Pages 110-116. PMID: 10442580.

[2] Ronenn Roubenoff, Virginia A. Hughes. "Sarcopenia: Current Concepts". *The Journals of Gerontology:* Series A, Volume 55, Issue 12, 1 December 2000, Pages M716-M724, https://doi.org/10.1093/gerona/55.12.M716

[3] Keller, K.; Engelhardt, M. "Strength and muscle mass loss with aging process. Age and strength loss". *Muscle, Ligaments, and Tendons Journal:* Oct-Dec 2013. Volume 3, Issue 4. Pages 346-350.

[4] Walston, J. "Sarcopenia in older adults". *Current Opinion in Rheumatology:* November 2012. Volume 24, Issue 6. Pages 623-627. doi: 10.1097/BOR.0b013e328358d59b

[5] Vetrano DL, Landi F, Volpato S, Corsonello A, Meloni E, Bernabei R, Onder G. "Association of Sarcopenia With Short- and Long-term Mortality in Older Adults Admitted to Acute Care Wards: Results From the CRIME Study". *The journals of Gerontology*: 2014. Series A, Biological sciences and medical sciences. DOI: 69.10.1093/gerona/glu034.

[6] Mangram, A.; Dzandu, J.; Harootunian, G.; et al. "Why Elderly Patients with Ground Level Falls Die Within 30 Days and Beyond?" *Journal of Gerontology and Geriatric Research:* April 2016. Volume 5, Issue 2. Pages 1-7. doi: 10.4172/2167-7182.1000289

[7] Shell Point Retirement Community. (August 13, 2012). *10 Shocking Statistics About Elderly Falls.* Retrieved from Shell Point Retirement Community: http://shellpoint.org/blog/2012/08/13/10-shocking-statistics-about-elderly-falls/

[8] Guin, Ursula K. Le. Lao Tzu: Tao Te Ching (p. 93). Shambhala. Kindle Edition.

[9] M. Izquierdo, K. Häkkinen, J. Ibañez, M. Garrues, A. Antón, A. Zúñiga, J. L. Larrión and E. M. Gorostiaga. "Effects of strength training on muscle power and serum hormones in middle-aged and older men." *The Journal of Applied Physiology:* Volume 90, Issue, 1 April 2001. Pages 1497-1507, https://doi.org/10.1152/jappl.2001.90.4.1497

[10] Kraemer WJ, Häkkinen K, Newton RU, Nindl BC, Volek JS, McCormick

M, Gotshalk LA, Gordon SE, Fleck SJ, Campbell WW, Putukian M, Evans WJ. "Effects of heavy-resistance training on hormonal response patterns in younger vs. older men." *The Journal of Applied Phyusiology*: Volume 87, Issue 3, 1 Sep 1999. Pages 982-992.
https://doi.org/10.1152/jappl.1999.87.3.982

[11] Bergland, Christopher (2013, January 22). *Cortisol: Why The 'Stress' Hormone is Public Enemy No. 1*. Retrieved from Psychology Today:
https://www.psychologytoday.com/blog/the-athletes-way/201301/cortisol-why-the-stress-hormone-is-public-enemy-no-1

[12] Kerksick, Chad M; Wilborn, Colin D; Campbell, Bill I; Roberts, Michael D; Rasmussen, Christopher J; Greenwood, Michael; Kreider, Richard B. "Early-Phase Adaptations to a Split-Body, Linear Periodization Resistance Training Program in College-Aged and Middle-Aged Men". *The Journal of Strength & Conditioning Research*: May 2009, Volume 23, Issue 3. Pages 962-971.
doi: 10.1519/JSC.0b013e3181a00baf

[13] ReportLinker Insight, 2017. *Out of Shape? Americans Turn to Exercise to Get Fit*. ReportLinker, 2017. Web. Nov 26, 2017.
https://www.reportlinker.com/insight/shape-americans-exercise-get-fit.html

[14] Organisation for Economic Co-operation and Development. (2017). *Obesity Update 2017*. Paris, France.

[15] Ryan, RM; Frederick, CM; Lepes, D; Rubio, N; Sheldon, KM. "Intrinsic Motivation and Exercise". *International Journal of Sport Psychology*: 1997, Vol 28, Issue 4. Pages 335-354.

[16] Ibid.

[17] Willink, J. (January 25, 2016). *Jocko Motivation (From Jocko Podcast)*. Retrieved from: Jocko Podcast:
https://www.youtube.com/watch?v=IdTMDpizis8

[18] Maxwell, John C.. Failing Forward: Turning Mistakes into Stepping Stones for Success (Kindle Location 114). Thomas Nelson. Kindle Edition.

[19] Wilson, K; Brookfield, D. "Effect of Goal Setting on Motivation and Adherence in a Six-Week Exercise Program". *International Journal of Sport and Exercise Physiology*: January 2009, Vol 7, Issue 1. Pages 89-100. DOI: 10.1080/1612197X.2009.9671894

[20] Dishman RK, Sallis JF. "Determinants and interventions for physical activity and exercise". In: Bouchard C, Shephard RJ, Stephens T, eds. *Physical activity, fitness and health: International proceedings and consensus statement*. Champaign, IL: *Human Kinetics*; 1994:Pages

214–238.

21 Kingston, A.; Robinson, L.; Booth, H.; Knapp, M; Jagger, C. "Projections of multi-morbidity in the older population in England to 2035: estimates from the Population Ageing and Care Simulation (PACSim) model". *Age and Ageing:* January 2018. Volume 0. Pages 1-7. doi: 10.1093/ageing/afx201

22 Sanders, Amy (February 9, 2016). *Don't Fall Off The "Fitness Cliff": How to Stick to Your New Year's Exercise Goals.* Retrieved from CBS News: https://www.cbsnews.com/news/dont-fall-off-the-fitness-cliff-stick-to-new-years-exercise-goals/

23 Morris, Z; Wooding S; Grant, J: "The answer is 17 years, what is the question: understanding time lags in translational research". *Journal of the Royal Society of Medicine*: Dec 16, 2011. Vol 104, Issue 12. Pages 510-520. DOI 10.1258/jrsm.2011.110180

24 Westcott, WL. "Resistance Training is Medicine: Effects of Strength Training on Health." *Current Sports Medicine Reports.* 2012 Jul-Aug;11(4):209-16. doi: 10.1249/JSR.0b013e31825dabb8.

25 Magee, A. (2016, March 14). *Why lifting is the new running for the over-40s.* Retrieved from Telegraph: http://www.telegraph.co.uk/health-fitness/body/why-lifting-is-the-new-running-for-the-over-40s/

26 Cavaliere, J. (n.d.). *How Much Weight to Lift to Build Muscle – You May Be Shocked.* Retrieved from Athlean-X: https://athleanx.com/blog/workout-tips/how-much-weight-to-lift-to-build-muscle

27 Cavaliere, J. (2016, May 14). *Workout Plan for Skinny Guys / Hardgainers (THIS BUILDS MUSCLE!).* Retrieved from Athlean-X YouTube Channel: https://www.youtube.com/watch?v=QVz0tXw7-FE

28 Swami, Radhanath. *The Journey Home* (p. 98). Insight Editions LLC. Kindle Edition.

29 *What is the strongest muscle in the human body?* (n.d.). *What is the strongest muscle in the human body?* Retrieved from Library of Congress: https://www.loc.gov/rr/scitech/mysteries/muscles.html

30 *Skeletal muscle fibers.* (n.d.). *Skeletal muscle fibers.* Retrieved from MediLexicon: http://www.medilexicon.com/dictionary/32960

31 *Skeletal Muscle Fiber Structure.* (n.d.) *Skeletal Muscle Fiber Structure.* Retrieved from University of California San Diego Muscle Physiology Home Page: http://muscle.ucsd.edu/musintro/myofiber.shtml

32 *Structure of Skeletal Muscle.* (n.d.) Retrieved from National Cancer Institute:

https://training.seer.cancer.gov/anatomy/muscular/structure.html

[33] Karp, J. R. "Muscle Fiber Types and Training". *Strength and Conditioning Journal*: October 2001. Volume 23, Issue 5. Pages 21-26.

[34] Ibid

[35] R Ricoy, J; Encinas, AR; Cabello, A; Madero, S; Arenas, J. "Histochemical study of the vastus lateralis muscle fibre types of athletes". *Journal of Physiology and Biochemistry*: April 1998. Volume 54. Pages 41-47.

[36] Qaisar, R; Bhaskaran, S; Van Remmen, H. "Muscle fiber type diversification during exercise and regeneration". *Free Radical Biology and Medicine:* September 2016. Volume 98. Pages 56-67. doi: 10.1016/j.freeradbiomed.2016.03.025

[37] Ibid

[38] Ibid

[39] Ibid

[40] Matthew 13:12

[41] Camera, D; Smiles, W; Hawley, J. "Exercise-induced skeletal muscle signaling pathways and human athletic performance". *Free Radical Biology and Medicine:* September 2016. Volume 98. Pages 131-143. doi: 10.1016/j.freeradbiomed.2016.02.007

[42] Van Mol, Peter (December 31, 2012). *The role of muscle damage in hypertrophy*. Retrieved from Muscle and Sports Science: http://muscleandsportsscience.com/the-role-of-muscle-damage-in-hypertrophy/

[43] How much physical activity do adults need? (n.d.) *How much physical activity do adults need?* Retrieved from US Centers for Disease Control: https://www.cdc.gov/physicalactivity/basics/adults/index.htm

[44] Schoenfeld, B; Ogborn, D; Krieger, J: "Effects of Resistance Training Frequency on Measures of Muscle Hypertrophy: A Systematic Review and Meta-Analysis". *Sports Medicine:* April 21, 2016. Volume 46, Issue 11. Pages 1689-1697.

[45] American College of Sports Medicine. "American College of Sports Medicine position stand. Progression models in resistance training for healthy adults". *Medicine and Science in Sports and Exercise*: March 2009. Volume 41, Issue 3. Pages 687-708. doi: 10.1249/MSS.0b013e3181915670

[46] McLester, J; Bishop, E; Guilliams, M.E. "Comparison of 1 Day and 3 Days Per Week of Equal-Volume Resistance Training in Experienced Subjects." Journal of Strength and Conditioning Research: August 2000. doi: 10.1097/00005768-199905001-00443

47 Gillam, M. "Effects of frequency of weight training on muscle strength enhancement". *The Journal of Sports Medicine and Physical Fitness*: 1982. Volume 21. Pages 432-436.

48 Schoenfeld, B. "The Mechanisms of Muscle Hypertrophy and Their Application to Resistance Training". *The Journal of Strength and Conditioning Research*: 2010. Volume 24, Issue 10. Pages 2857–2872.

49 Bloomer, R; Ives, J. "Varying Neural and Hypertrophic Influences in a Strength Program". *Strength and Conditioning Journal*: April 2000. Volume 22, Number 2. Pages 30-35.

50 Ferrugia, J. (n.d.). *How Long Should Your Workout Last if You Want to Build Muscle and Get Ripped?* Retrieved from JasonFerrugia.com: http://jasonferruggia.com/how-long-should-your-workout-last/

51 Holm, L; Reitelsefer; et al. "Changes in muscle size and MHC composition in response to resistance exercise with heavy and light loading intensity". *Journal of Applied Physiology:* Nov 1, 2008. Volume 105, Issue 5. Pages 1454-1461. doi: 10.1152/japplphysiol.90538.2008

52 Schoenfeld, B. "Is There a Minimum Intensity Threshold for Resistance Training-Induced Hypertrophic Adaptations?" *Sports Medicine*: December 2013. Volume 43, Issue 12. Pages 1297-1288. doi: 10.1007/s40279-013-0088-z

53 American College of Sports Medicine. "American College of Sports Medicine position stand. Progression models in resistance training for healthy adults". *Medicine and Science in Sports and Exercise*: March 2009. Volume 41, Issue 3. Pages 687-708. doi: 10.1249/MSS.0b013e3181915670

54 Schoenfeld, B. "The Mechanisms of Muscle Hypertrophy and Their Application to Resistance Training". *The Journal of Strength and Conditioning Research*: 2010. Volume 24, Issue 10. Pages 2857–2872.

55 Pakulski, B. (n.d.) *Foundational Training for Muscle-Building Success (Part 3)*. Retrieved from Ben Pakulski Athletics: http://www.benpakulski.com/mi40-university/foundational-training-muscle-building-success-part-3/

56 Schoenfeld, B. (November 25, 2015). *The New Science of Time Under Tension*. Retrieved from T-Nation: https://www.t-nation.com/training/new-science-of-time-under-tension

57 Pakulski, B. (nd.d). *Ben Pakulski: Chest Expansion*. Retrieved from FlexOnline: https://www.flexonline.com/ben-pakulski-chest-expansion

58 Wilson, D. J. (2017, September 13). *Time Under Tension for Muscle Growth*. Retrieved from The Muscle PhD: https://themusclephd.com/time-tension-muscle-growth/

[59] Burd, N; et al. "Muscle Time Under Tension During Resistance Exercise Stimulates Differential Muscle Protein Sub-Fractional Synthetic Responses in Men". *The Journal of Physiology:* January 15, 2012. Volume 590, Part 2. Pages 351-362. doi: 10.1113/jphysiol.2011.221200

[60] Nóbrega, S.; Ugrinowitsch, C.; Pintanel, L.; Barcelos, C.; Libardi, C. "Effect of Resistance Training to Muscle Failure vs. Volitional Interruption at High- and Low-Intensities on Muscle Mass and Strength." *The Journal of Strength and Conditioning Research:* January 2018. Volume 32, Issue 1. Pages 162-169. doi: 10.1519/JSC.0000000000001787

[61] Bird, S; Marino, F; et al. "Designing Resistance Training Programmes to Enhance Muscular Fitness". *Sports Medicine*: February 2005. Volume 35, Issue 10. Pages 841-851. doi: 10.2165/00007256-200535100-00002

[62] Kraemer, W; et al. "Endogenous Anabolic Hormonal and Growth Factor Responses to Heavy Resistance Exercise in Males and Females". *International Journal of Sports Medicine*: April 1991. Volume 12, Issue 2. Pages 228-235. doi: 10.1055/s-2007-1024673

[63] Bird, S; Marino, F; et al. "Designing Resistance Training Programmes to Enhance Muscular Fitness". *Sports Medicine*: February 2005. Volume 35, Issue 10. Pages 841-851. doi: 10.2165/00007256-200535100-00002

[64] Baechle, T & Earle, R. (Eds.). (2008). *Essentials of Strength Training and Conditioning: Third Edition*. Champaign, IL: Human Kinetics.

[65] Pakulski, B. (n.d.) *Is your Rep Speed KILLING your gains?* Retrieved from Ben Pakulski Athletics: http://www.benpakulski.com/uncategorized/rep-speed-killing-gains/

[66] Gallwey, W. Timothy. *The Inner Game of Tennis: The Classic Guide to the Mental Side of Peak Performance* (p. 2). Random House Publishing Group. Kindle Edition.

[67] Murphy, Michael. In the Zone: Transcendent Experience in Sports (p. 75). Open Road Media. Kindle Edition.

[68] Gallwey, W. Timothy. *The Inner Game of Tennis: The Classic Guide to the Mental Side of Peak Performance* (p. 7). Random House Publishing Group. Kindle Edition.

[69] Lipsyte, R. *Sportsworld*. (1975). New York: Quadrangle/New York Times Book Co.

[70] Csikszentmihalyi, M. *Flow: The Psychology of Optimal Experience* (p. 3). HarperCollins Publishers. Kindle Edition.

[71] Gallwey, W. Timothy. *The Inner Game of Tennis: The Classic Guide to the Mental Side of Peak Performance* (p. 43). Random House Publishing

Group. Kindle Edition.

[72] Napoli, N. (March 1, 2018). Music Boosts Exercise Time During Cardiac Stress Testing. Retrieved from American College of Cardiology: http://www.acc.org/about-acc/press-releases/2018/02/27/12/01/music-boosts-exercise-time-during-cardiac-stress-testing

[73] Billat, LV. "Interval Training for Performance: A Scientific and Empirical Practice". *Sports Medicine:* January 2001. Volume 31, Issue 1. Pages 13-31.

[74] Carey, D. "Quantifying Differences in the "Fat Burning" Zone and the Aerobic Zone: Implications for Training". *The Journal of Strength and Conditioning Research:* October 2009. Volume 23, Issue 7. Pages 2090-2095. doi: 10.1519/JSC.0b013e3181bac5c5

[75] Ibid

[76] Dieter, Brad. (October 6, 2015). *Fat and Carbohydrate Utilization During Exercise.* Retrieved from Science Driven Nutrition: http://sciencedrivennutrition.com/fat-and-carbohydrate-utilization-during-exercise/

[77] Melzer, K. "Carbohydrate and fat utilization during rest and physical activity". *E-SPEN, the European e-Journal of Clinical Nutrition and Metabolism:* April 2011. Volume 6, Issue 2. Pages e45-e52. doi: 10.1016/j.eclnm.2011.01.005

[78] National Council on Strength and Fitness. (n.d.). *Relationship between Percent HR Max and Percent VO$_2$max.* Retrieved from National Council on Strength and Fitness: https://www.ncsf.org/pdf/ceu/relationship_between_percent_hr_max_and_percent_vo2_max.pdf

[79] Melzer, K. "Carbohydrate and fat utilization during rest and physical activity". *E-SPEN, the European e-Journal of Clinical Nutrition and Metabolism:* April 2011. Volume 6, Issue 2. Pages e45-e52. doi: 10.1016/j.eclnm.2011.01.005

[80] Ibid.

[81] Bird, B. (July 18, 2017). *Why Do Our Bodies Burn Carbohydrates Before Fat?* Retrieved from Livestrong.com: https://www.livestrong.com/article/467835-why-do-our-bodies-burn-carbohydrates-before-fat/

[82] Poliquin Group Editorial Staff. (February 19, 2014). *Eleven Myths and Facts About How the Body Burns Fat.* Retrieved from Poliquin Group: http://main.poliquingroup.com/ArticlesMultimedia/Articles/PrinterFriendly.aspx?ID=1122&lang=en

[83] Benson, Roy. Heart Rate Training (Kindle Locations 864-866). Human

Kinetics - A. Kindle Edition.

[84] *The ATP-PC System*. (n.d.) *The ATP-PC System*. Retrieved from: PTDirect: https://www.ptdirect.com/training-design/anatomy-and-physiology/the-atp-pc-system

[85] Roth, S. (January 23, 2006). *Why Does Lactic Acid Build Up in Muscles? And Why Does It Cause Soreness?* Retrieved from Scientific American: https://www.scientificamerican.com/article/why-does-lactic-acid-buil/

[86] Carey, D. "Quantifying Differences in the "Fat Burning" Zone and the Aerobic Zone: Implications for Training". *The Journal of Strength and Conditioning Research:* October 2009. Volume 23, Issue 7. Pages 2090-2095. doi: 10.1519/JSC.0b013e3181bac5c5

[87] Ibid.

[88] Romijn, JA; et al. "Regulation of endogenous fat and carbohydrate metabolism in relation to exercise intensity and duration". *American Journal of Physiology*: September 1993. Volume 3, Part 1. Pages E380-391. doi: 10.1152/ajpendo.1993.265.3.E380

[89] Carey, D. "Quantifying Differences in the "Fat Burning" Zone and the Aerobic Zone: Implications for Training". *The Journal of Strength and Conditioning Research:* October 2009. Volume 23, Issue 7. Pages 2090-2095. doi: 10.1519/JSC.0b013e3181bac5c5

[90] Sock Dock. (n.d.). *Sock Dock Training Part I. Aerobic Activity is the Foundation to Your Health AND Fitness*. Retrieved from Sock Doc: http://sock-doc.com/aerobic-vs-anaerobic-exercise/

[91] Norris, R.; et al. "The effects of aerobic and anaerobic training on fitness, blood pressure, and psychological stress and well-being". *Journal of Psychosomatic Research*: 1990. Volume 34, Issue 4. Pages 367-375. doi: 10.1016/0022-3999(90)90060-H

[92] Ratamess, N; et al. "Acute Resistance Exercise Performance is Negatively Impacted by Prior Aerobic Endurance Exercise". *Journal of Strength and Conditioning Research:* October 2016. Volume 30, Issue 10. Pages 2667-2681. doi: 10.1519/JSC.0000000000001548

[93] Rahnama, S. (October 17, 2005). *Timing is Everything: Why the Duration and Order of Your Exercise Matters*. Retrieved from University of Michigan MedFitness: http://umich.edu/~medfit/resistancetraining/timingiseverything101705.html

[94] Wilson, D. J. (2017, November 16). *Do's & Don'ts of Cardio & Fat Loss*. Retrieved from The Muscle PhD: https://themusclephd.com/cardio-fat-loss/

[95] Wilson, D. J. (May 29, 2017). *How Does HIIT Get You Jacked and Shredded?*. Retrieved from The Muscle PhD: https://themusclephd.com/how-does-HIIT-get-you-jacked-shredded/

[96] Herbert, P; et al. "HIIT produces increases in muscle power and free testosterone in male masters athletes". *Endocrine Connections*: 21 July 2017. Volume 6, Number 7. Pages 430-436.

[97] Laurent, M; et al. "Sex-specific responses to self-paced, high-intensity interval training with variable recovery periods". Journal of Strength and Conditioning Research: April 2014. Volume 4. Pages 920-927.

[98] Kelso, T. (n.d.). *How to Choose the Proper Work and Rest Periods When Interval Training*. Retrieved from Breaking Muscle: https://breakingmuscle.com/fitness/how-to-choose-the-proper-work-and-rest-periods-when-interval-training

[99] Tabata, I; Motohiko, M; Futoshi, O. "Effects of moderate-intensity endurance and high-intensity intermittent training on anaerobic capacity and VO(2max)". *Medicine and Science in Sports and Exercise*: October 1996. Volume 28, Issue 10. Pages 1327-1330.

[100] Foster, C; et al. "The Effects of High Intensity Interval Training vs Steady State Training on Aerobic and Anaerobic Capacity". *Journal of Sports Science and Medicine:* December 2015. Volume 14, Issue 4. Pages 747-755.

[101] Ibid.

[102] Gibala, M; Little, JP; et al. "Short-term interval versus traditional endurance training: similar initial adaptations in human skeletal muscle and exercise performance." *Journal of Physiology:* September 2006. Volume 15, Issue 575 (Part 3). Pages 901-911. doi: 10.1113/jphysiol.2006.112094

[103] Marker, C. (n.d.). *How Tabata Really Works: What the Research Says*. Retrieved from Breaking Muscle: https://breakingmuscle.com/fitness/how-tabata-really-works-what-the-research-says

[104] Hazell, TJ; Oliver, TD; et al. "Two minutes of sprint-interval exercise elicits 24-hr oxygen consumption similar to that of 30 min of continuous exercise". *International Journal of Sport Nutrition and Exercise Metabolism:* August 2012. Volume 4. Pages 276-283.

[105] Erikssen G, Liestø K, Bjørnholt J, et al. "Changes in physical fitness and changes in mortality". *Lancet:* September 1998. Volume 352. Pages 759-762.

[106] Lee IM, Hsieh CC, Paffenbarger RS Jr. *Exercise intensity and longevity in men. The Harvard Alumni Health Study:* Journal of the

American Medical Association: April 19, 1995. Volume 273. Pages 1179-1184.

[107] Ballantyne, C. January 2, 2009. *Does Exercise Make You Healthier?* Retrieved from Scientific American: https://www.scientificamerican.com/article/does-exercise-really-make/

[108] Fontana, L; Partridge, L. "Promoting Health and Longevity through Diet: From Model Organisms to Humans". *Cell:* March 26, 2015. Pages 106-118. doi: 10.1016/j.cell.2015.02.020

[109] Odebunmi, O. (September 11, 2017). *Exercise Programs for Middle-Aged Men.* Retrieved from Livestrong: https://www.livestrong.com/article/404510-exercise-programs-for-middle-age-men/

[110] Deida, David. The Way of the Superior Man: A Spiritual Guide to Mastering the Challenges of Women, Work, and Sexual Desire (p. 189). Sounds True. Kindle Edition.

[111] Centro Nacional de Investigaciones Oncologicas. (July 3, 2014). *Size of the human genome reduced to 19,000 genes.* Retrieved from Science Daily: https://www.sciencedaily.com/releases/2014/07/140703112830.htm

[112] Prestes, J.; De Lima, C.; et al. "Comparison of Linear and Reverse Linear Periodization Effects on Maximal Strength and Body Composition". *Journal of Strength and Conditioning Research:* January 2009. Volume 23, Number 1. Pages 266-274.

[113] Kerksick, C.; Wilborn, C.; Campbell, B.; et al. "Early-Phase Adaptations to a Split-Body Linear Periodization Program in College-Aged and Middle-Aged Men". *Journal of Strength and Conditioning Research:* May 2009. Volume 23, Number 3. Pages 963-971.

[114] McDole, J. (April 7, 2011). *Linear, Undulating, and Nonlinear Programming: Which to Choose?* Retrieved from Elitelifts: https://www.elitefts.com/education/training/powerlifting/linear-undulating-and-nonlinear-programming-which-to-choose/

[115] Kerksick, C.; Wilborn, C.; Campbell, B.; et al. "Early-Phase Adaptations to a Split-Body Linear Periodization Program in College-Aged and Middle-Aged Men". *Journal of Strength and Conditioning Research:* May 2009. Volume 23, Number 3. Pages 963-971.

[116] Simão, R.; Spineti, J.; Freitas de Salles, B.; et al. "Comparison Between Nonlinear and Linear Periodized Resistance Training: Hypertrophic and Strength Effects". *Journal of Strength and Conditioning Research:* May 2012. Volume 26, Number 5. Pages 1389-1395.

[117] Rhea, M.; Ball, S.; Phillips, W.; Burkett, L. "A Comparison of Linear and Daily Undulating Periodized Programs with Equated

Volume and Intensity for Strength". *Journal of Strength and Conditioning Research:* May 2002. Volume 16, Issue 2. Pages 250-255.

[118] Simão, R.; Spineti, J.; Freitas de Salles, B.; et al. "Comparison Between Nonlinear and Linear Periodized Resistance Training: Hypertrophic and Strength Effects". *Journal of Strength and Conditioning Research:* May 2012. Volume 26, Number 5. Pages 1389-1395.

[119] Pagel, J. (n.d.). Daily Undulating Periodization Strategy (DUP) Training. Retrieved from AskMen: https://www.askmen.com/sports/bodybuilding/daily-undulating-periodization-dup-training.html

[120] Wang, C. (April 5, 2016). How a Health Nut Created the World's Biggest Fitness Trend. Retrieved from CNBC: https://www.cnbc.com/2016/04/05/how-crossfit-rode-a-single-issue-to-world-fitness-domination.html

[121] Kamb, S. (n.d.) *A Beginner's Guide to Crossfit.* Retrieved from Nerd Fitness: https://www.nerdfitness.com/blog/a-beginners-guide-to-crossfit/

[122] The Business of CrossFit: An Update on New Market Research. (March 13, 2017). The Business of CrossFit: An Update on New Market Research. Retrieved from Rally Fitness: https://rallyfitness.com/blogs/news/the-business-of-crossfit-an-update-on-new-market-research-2017

[123] *What is CrossFit?* (n.d.) *What is CrossFit?.* Retrieved from CrossFit: https://www.crossfit.com/what-is-crossfit

[124] Ibid.

[125] Paine, J.; Uptgaft, J.; Wylie, R. "CrossFit Study". *Comprehensive Soldier Fitness, Command and General Staff College:* May 2010.

[126] Murawska-Cialowicz, E.; Wojna, J.; Zuwala-Jagiello, J. "Crossfit training changes brain-derived neurotrophic factor and irisin levels at rest, after wingate and progressive tests, and improves aerobic capacity and body composition of young physically active men and women." *Journal of Physiology and Pharmacology:* December 2015, Volume 66, Issue 6. Pages 811-821.

[127] OfficialTheNX. November 5, 2017. *The Problem With CrossFit.* Retrieved from: https://www.youtube.com/watch?v=YAuc-LSS6iQ

[128] TigerFitness. October 28, 2015. *Why CrossFit is losing its popularity.* Retrieved from: https://www.youtube.com/watch?time_continue=2&v=cM9wiCCdFi4

[129] Alfonsi, S. (May 10, 2015). King of CrossFit. Retrieved from CBS

News: https://www.cbsnews.com/news/crossfit-creator-greg-glassman-60-minutes/

[130] Hak, P.; Hodzovic, E.; Hickey, B. "The nature and prevalence of injury during CrossFit training." *Journal of Strength and Conditioning Research:* November 2013. doi: 10.1519/JSC.0000000000000318

[131] McCarty, P. (n.d.) *The Great Injury Debate: Is CrossFit Dangerous? We May Never Know.* Retrieved from Breaking Muscle: https://breakingmuscle.com/fitness/the-great-injury-debate-is-crossfit-dangerous-we-may-never-know

[132] Pyfferoen, B. (May 30, 2017). *Pec Tears at Regionals ... 36!* Retrieved from Barbell Spin: http://thebarbellspin.com/functional-fitness/pec-tears-at-regionals-23-and-counting/

[133] Hak, P.; Hodzovic, E.; Hickey, B. "The nature and prevalence of injury during CrossFit training." *Journal of Strength and Conditioning Research:* November 2013. doi: 10.1519/JSC.0000000000000318

[134] Downey, J. "Parenting practices related to positive eating, physical activity and sedentary behaviors in children: A qualitative exploration of strategies used by parents to navigate the obesigenic environment". *Graduate Theses and Dissertations:* 2014. 13964. http://lib.dr.iastate.edu/etd/13964

[135] Lunden, J.; Winick, M. (2004) *Growing Up Healthy: Protecting Your Child from Diseases Now Through Adulthood:* New York, NY. Atria (Simon and Schuster)

[136] Marsiglio, W.; Amato, O.; Day, R.; Lamb, M. "Scholarship on Fatherhood in the 1990's and Beyond". *Journal of Marriage and the Family:* November 2000. Volume 62. Pages 1173-1191.

[137] Aurelius, Marcus. Stoic Six Pack - Meditations of Marcus Aurelius, Golden Sayings, Fragments and Discourses of Epictetus, Letters From A Stoic and The Enchiridion (Illustrated) (p. 350). Unknown. Kindle Edition.

[138] Robbins, T. (n.d.). *Progress Equal Happiness.* Retrieved from Robbins Research: https://www.tonyrobbins.com/leadership-impact/feel-good-now/

[139] Godin, Seth. The Dip: A Little Book That Teaches You When to Quit (and When to Stick) (p. 17). Penguin Publishing Group. Kindle Edition.

[140] Godin, Seth. The Dip: A Little Book That Teaches You When to Quit (and When to Stick) (pp. 23-24). Penguin Publishing Group. Kindle Edition.

[141] Bloomer, R.; Ives, J. "Varying Neural and Hypertrophic Influences in a Strength Program". *Strength and Conditioning Journal:* April 2000.

Volume 22, Number 2. Pages 30-35.

[142] Spriet, L.; Gibala, M. "Nutritional strategies to influence adaptations to training." *Journal of Sports Sciences:* 2004. Volume 22, Issue 1. Pages 127-141.

[143] Parsley, K. (June 3, 2017). Why Should I Care About Sleep? Retrieved from DocParsley.com: http://www.docparsley.com/2017/06/why-should-i-care-about-sleep/

[144] Sullivan,Alycia N; Lachman,Margie E. "Behavior Change with Fitness Technology in Sedentary Adults: A Review of the Evidence for Increasing Physical Activity". *Frontiers in Public Health:*.Jan 11, 2017. doi: 10.3389/fpubh.2016.00289

[145] Coutinho, T.; Goel, K.; Corrêa de Sá, D.; et al. "Combining Body Mass Index With Measures of Central Obesity in the Assessment of Mortality in Subjects With Coronary Disease: Role of "Normal Weight Central Obesity". *Journal of the American College of Cardiology:* February 2013. Volume 61, Issue 5. Pages 553-560. doi: 10.1016/j.jacc.2012.10.035

[146] Shiwei, S.; Lu, Y.; Qi, H; et al. "Waist-to-height ratio is an effective indicator for comprehensive cardiac health." *Scientific Reports:* February 2017. Volume 7, Article Number 43046. doi: 10.1038/srep43046

[147] Weeden, J.; Sabini, J. "Physical Attractiveness and Health in Western Societies: A Review". *Psychological Bulletin:* 2005. Volume 13, Number 5. Pages 635-653.

[148] Goodarz, D.; Lawes, C.; Vander Hoorn, S.; et al. "Global and regional mortality from ischaemic heart disease and stroke attributable to higher-than-optimum blood glucose concentration: comparative risk assessment". Lancet: November 11-17, 2006. Volume 368, Issue 9549. Pages 1651-1659. doi: 10.1016/S0140-6736(06)69700-6

[149] Jee, S.; Ohrr, H.; Sull, J. "Fasting Serum Glucose Level and Cancer Risk in Korean Men and Women". *Journal of the American Medical Association:* January 12, 2005. Volume 293, Issue 2. Pages 194-202. doi: 10.1001/jama.293.2.194

[150] De la Monte, S.; Wands, J. "Alzheimer's Disease Is Type 3 Diabetes – Evidence Reviewed." *Journal of Diabetic Science and Technology:* November 2008. Volume 2, Issue 6. Pages 1101-1113. doi: 10.1177/193229680800200619

[151] Zheng, F.; Yan, L.; Yang, Z.; Zhong, B.; Xie, W. "HbA$_{1c}$, diabetes, and cognitive decline: the English Longitudinal Study of Ageing". *Diabetologia:* January 25, 2018. Pages 1-10. doi: 10.1007/s00125-017-4541-7

[152] Moubarac, J.; Bortoletto Martins, A. "Consumption of ultra-processed foods and likely impact on human health. Evidence from Canada." *Public Health Nutrition:* December 2013. Volume 16, Issue 12. Pages 2240-2248. doi: 10.1017/S1368980012005009

[153] Heid, M. (April 24, 2015). Which One's More Important: Diet or Exercise? Retrieved from Prevention.com: https://www.prevention.com/weight-loss/diet-vs-exercise

[154] McDonald's Nutrition Calculator. (n.d.), McDonald's Nutrition Calculator. Retrieved from McDonalds.com: https://www.mcdonalds.com/us/en-us/about-our-food/nutrition-calculator.html

[155] Explore Our Menu. (n.d.) Explore Our Menu. Retrieved from Starbucks.com: https://www.starbucks.com/menu/catalog/nutrition?food=hot-breakfast#view_control=nutrition

[156] Eslami, S.; Taherzadeh, Z.; Schultz, M.; Abu-Hanna, A. "Glucose variability measures and their effect on mortality: a systemic review". *Intensive Care Medicine:* April 2011. Volume 37, Issue 4. Pages 583-593.

[157] Berg, J.; Tymoczko, J.; Stryer, L. (2002) *Biochemistry: Fifth Edition.* New York, NY: W.H. Freeman and Company.

[158] Myosins (n.d.) Myosins. Retrieved from US National Library of Medicine – Genetics Home Reference: https://ghr.nlm.nih.gov/primer/genefamily/myosins

[159] Atherton, P.; Smith, K. "Muscle protein synthesis in response to nutrition and exercise". The Journal of Physiology: Mar 1, 2012. Volume 590, Part 5. Pages 1049-1057.

[160] Phillips, S. "Dietary protein requirements and adaptive advantages in athletes." *British Journal of Nutrition:* August 2012. Volume 108, Supplement S2. Pages S158-S167. doi: 10.1017/S0007114512002516

[161] Helms, E.; Rowlands, D.; Zinn, C.; Brown, S. "A Systematic Review of Dietary Protein During Caloric Restriction in Resistance Trained Lean Athletes: A Case for Higher Intakes." *International Journal of Sport Nutrition and Exercise Metabolism:* October 2013. Volume 24. Pages 127-138. doi: 10.1123/ijsnem.2013-0054

[162] Henselmans, M. (October 28, 2015). Eric Helms and protein:A research review. Retrieved from BayesianBodybuilding.com: https://bayesianbodybuilding.com/eric-helms-protein/

[163] Roasted Chicken Breast, With Skin. (n.d.). Roasted Chicken Breast, With Skin. Retrieved from CalorieKing.com:

http://www.calorieking.com/foods/calories-in-chicken-roasted-chicken-breast-with-skin_f-ZmlkPTY4MzEz.html

164 Meijer True Goodness: Grass Fed Ground Beef, 90% Lean 10% Fat, raw. (n.d.) Meijer True Goodness: Grass Fed Ground Beef, 90% Lean 10% Fat, raw. Retrieved from CalorieKing.com: http://www.calorieking.com/foods/calories-in-beef-true-goodness-grass-fed-ground-beef-90-lean-10-fat-raw_f-ZmlkPTEwMDMyMDc2.html

165 Daley, C.; Abbott, A.; Doyle, P.; Nader, G.; Larson, S. "A review of fatty acid profiles and antioxidant content in grass-fed and grain-fed beef". *BMC Nutrition Journal:* March 10, 2010. Volume 9, Issue 10. doi: 10.1186/1475-2891-9-10

166 Whey Protein. (n.d.) Whey Protein. Retrieved from Examine.com: https://examine.com/supplements/whey-protein/

167 Stark, M.; Lumaszuk, J. "Protein timing and its effects on muscular hypertrophy and strength in individuals engaged in weight-training". *Journal of the International Society of Sports Nutrition:* December 14, 2012. Volume 9, Issue 54. doi: 10.1186/1550-2783-9-54

168 Walker, T.; Smith, J.; Herrera, M.; Lebegue, B.; Pinchak, A.; Fischer, J. "The influence of 8 weeks of whey-protein and leucine supplementation on physical and cognitive performance." *International Journal Of Sport Nutrition And Exercise Metabolism:* October 2010. Volume 20, Issue 5. Pages 409-417.

169 Chaudhuri, J. (n.d.) Ketone Body Metabolism. Retrieved from SRM University: http://www.srmuniv.ac.in/sites/default/files/files/KETONEBODYMETABOLISM.pdf

170 Roberts, M. (March 12, 2017). The IRONMAN Guide to Ketosis. Retrieved from NourishBalanceThrive.com: http://www.nourishbalancethrive.com/blog/2017/03/12/ironman-guide-ketosis/

171 Willett, B. (October 3, 2017). The Advantages and Disadvantages of Ketosis. Retrieved from LiveStrong.com: https://www.livestrong.com/article/492485-the-advantages-disadvantages-of-ketosis/

172 What is the Keto Flu and How do You Cure it? (n.d.) What is the Keto Flu and How do You Cure it? Retrieved from KettleAndFire.com: https://blog.kettleandfire.com/keto-flu/

173 Scott-Dixon, K.; Kollias, H. (n.d.) The Ketogenic Diet: Does it live up to the hype? Retrieved from PrecisionNutrition.com: https://www.precisionnutrition.com/ketogenic-diet

[174] Paleo. (n.d.) Paleo. Retrieved from Dictionary.com: http://www.dictionary.com/browse/paleo

[175] Wolf, R. (n.d.) What is the Paleo Diet? Retrieved from RobbWolf.com: https://robbwolf.com/what-is-the-paleo-diet/

[176] Durant, J. (2013). *The Paleo Manifesto: Ancient Wisdom For Lifelong Health*. New York City, NY: Penguin Random House Company.

[177] Frassetto, L.; Schloetter, M.; Mietus-Snyder, M.; Morris, R.; Sebastian, A. "Metabolic and physiologic improvements from consuming a paleolithic, hunter-gatherer type diet". *European Journal of Clinical Nutrition:* 2009. Volume 63. Pages 947-955. doi: 10.1038/ejcn.2015.193

[178] Masharani, U; et al. "Metabolic and physiologic effects from consuming a hunter-gatherer (Paleolithic)-type diet in type 2 diabetes". *European Journal of Clinical Nutrition:* 2015. Volume 69. Pages 944-948. doi: 10.1038/ejcn.2015.39

[179] Manheimer, E.; Van Zuuren, E.; Fedorowicz, Z.; Hanno, P. "Paleolithic nutrition for metabolic syndrome: systematic review and meta-analysis". *The American Journal of Clinical Nutrition:* October 2015. Volume 102, Issue 4. Pages 922-932. doi: 10.3945/ajcn.115.113613

[180] Dugdale, M. (January 15, 2015). The Food Philosophy of an IFBB Pro. Retrieved from EliteFTS.com: https://www.elitefts.com/education/the-food-philosophy-of-an-ifbb-pro/

[181] Smith, M.; Trexler, E.; Sommer, A.; Starkoff, E.; Devor, S. "Unrestricted Paleolithic Diet is Associated with Unfavorable Changes to Blood Lipids in Healthy Subjects". *International Journal of Exercise Science:* 2014. Volume 7, Issue 2. Pages 128-139.

[182] Jabr, F. (June 3, 2013). How to Really Eat Like a Hunter-Gatherer: Why the Paleo Diet is Half-Baked. Retrieved from ScientificAmerican.com: https://www.scientificamerican.com/article/why-paleo-diet-half-baked-how-hunter-gatherer-really-eat/

[183] Paleo Diet. (n.d.) Paleo Diet. Retrieved from US News and World Report: https://health.usnews.com/best-diet/paleo-diet

[184] Mediterranean Diet. (n.d.) Mediterranean Diet. Retrieved from US News and World Report: https://health.usnews.com/best-diet/mediterranean-diet

[185] Willett, W.C.; Sacks, F.; et al. "Mediterranean diet pyramid: a cultural model for healthy eating". *The American Journal of Clinical Nutrition:* June 1, 1995. Volume 61, Issue 6. Pages 1402S-1406S. doi:

10.1093/ajcn/61.6.1402S

[186] Knoops, K.; De Groot, L.; Kromhout, D.; et al. "Mediterranean Diet, Lifestyle Factors, and 10-Year Mortality in Elderly European Men and Women". *Journal of the American Medical Assocation:* September 2004. Volume 292, Issue 12. Pages 1433-1439. doi: 10.1001/jama.292.12.1433

[187] Estruch, R.; Ros, E.; et al. "Primary Prevention of Cardiovascular Disease With a Mediterranean Diet". *The New England Journal of Medicine:* April 2013. Volume 1368. Pages 1279-1290. doi: 10.1056/NEJMoa1200303

[188] Scarmeas, N.; Stern, Y.; et al. "Mediterranean Diet and Risk for Alzheimer's Disease". *Annals of Neurology:* June 2006. Volume 59, Issue 6. Pages 912-921. doi: 10.1002/ana.20854

[189] Antonio, J.; Kalman, D, Stout, J.; et al. (2008). *Eating to Improve Body Composition.* Totowa, NJ: Humana Press.

[190] Lennon, D. (November 19, 2014). The Ridiculously Simple Guide to Sustainable Fat Loss. Retrieved from Sigma Nutrition : http://sigmanutrition.com/the-ridiculously-simple-guide-to-sustainable-results/

[191] **Retail sales of vitamins & nutritional supplements in the United States from 2000 to 2017 (in billion US dollars). (n.d.). Retail sales of vitamins & nutritional supplements in the United States from 2000 to 2017 (in billion US dollars). Retrieved from Statista.com: https://www.statista.com/statistics/235801/retail-sales-of-vitamins-and-nutritional-supplements-in-the-us/**

[192] Cooper, L. (May 19, 2017). Liver Damage From Supplements Is on the Rise: Green-tea extract and bodybuilding pills pose a particular risk, study finds. Retrieved from ConsumerReports.org: https://www.consumerreports.org/health/liver-damage-from-supplements-is-on-the-rise/

[193] Krishna, YR; Mittal, V; et al. "Acute liver failure caused by 'fat burners' and dietary supplements: A case report and literature review". *Canadian Journal of Gastroenterology:* March 2011. Volume 25, Issue 3. Page 157-160.

[194] Cohen, P. "American Roulette – Contaminated Dietary Supplements". *New England Journal of Medicine:* October 2009. Volume 361. Pages 1523-1525. doi: 10.1056/NEJMp0904768

[195] Jenkins, M. (1998) Creatine Supplementation in Athletes: Review. Retrieved from Rice University:

http://www.rice.edu/~jenky/sports/creatine.html

[196] The ATP-PC System. (n.d.) The ATP-PC System. Retrieved from PTDirect.com: https://www.ptdirect.com/training-design/anatomy-and-physiology/the-atp-pc-system

[197] Balsom, P.; Söderlund, K.; Ekblom, B. "Creatine in Humans with Special Reference to Creatine Supplementation." *Sports Medicine:* 1994. Volume 18, Issue 4. Pages 268-280.

[198] Buford, T.; Kreider, R.; et al. "International Society of Sports Nutrition position stand: creatine supplementation and exercise". *Journal of the International Society of Sports Nutrition:* August 2007. Volume 4, Issue 6. doi: 10.1186/1550-2783-4-6

[199] Balsom, P.; Söderlund, K.; Ekblom, B. "Creatine in Humans with Special Reference to Creatine Supplementation." *Sports Medicine:* 1994. Volume 18, Issue 4. Pages 268-280.

[200] Smith, S.; Montain, S.; Matott, R.; et al. "Creatine supplementation and age influence muscle metabolism during exercise". *Journal of Applied Physiology:* October 1998. Volume 85, Issue 4. Pages 1349-1356. doi: 10.1152/jappl.1998.85.4.1349

[201] Sari-Sarraf, V.; Amirsasan, R.; Sheikholeslami-Vatani, D.; Faraji, H. "The effect of creatine monohydrate supplementation on apoptosis at acute resistance exercise in middle-aged men". *Iranian Journal of Nutrition Sciences and Food Technology:* 2016. Volume 11, Number 4. Pages 47-54.

[202] Becque, D.; Lochmann, J.; Melrose, D. "Effects of oral creatine supplementation on muscular strength and body composition". *Medicine and Science in Sports and Exercise:* March 2000. Volume 32, Issue 3. Pages 654-658.

[203] Dorrell, H.; Gee, T.; Middleton, G. "An Update on Effects of Creatine Supplementation on Performance: A Review". *Sports Nutrition and Therapy:* March 2016. Volume 1, Issue 1. doi: 10.4172/snt.1000107

[204] Jeronimo, D.; Germano, M.; Fiorante, L.; et al. "Caffeine Potentiates the Ergogenic Effects of Creatine". *Journal of Physiology Online:* December 2017. Volume 20, Number 6. Pages 66-77.

[205] Smith, R.; Agharkar, A.; Gonzalez, E. "A review of creatine supplementation in age-related diseases: more than a supplement for athletes". *F1000 Research:* September 2014. Volume 3, Issue 222. doi: 10.12688/f1000research.5218.1

[206] Rae, C.; Digney, A.; McEwan, S.; Bates, T. "Oral creatine monohydrate supplementation improves brain performance: a double-blind, placebo-controlled, cross-over trial". *Proceedings of the Royal Society B: Biological Sciences:* October 2003. Volume 270, Issue 1529.

Pages 2147-2150. doi: 10.1098/rspb.2003.2492

[207] Summary of Beta-Alanine. (n.d.). Summary of Beta-Alanine. Retrieved from Examine.com: https://examine.com/supplements/beta-alanine/

[208] The Anaerobic Glycolytic System (fast glycolysis). (n.d.) The Anaerobic Glycolytic System (fast glycolysis). Retrieved from PTDirect.com: https://www.ptdirect.com/training-design/anatomy-and-physiology/the-anaerobic-glycolytic-system-fast-glycolysis

[209] Artioli, G.; Gualano, B.; et al. "The Role of β-alanine Supplementation on Muscle Carnosine and Exercise Performance". *Medicine and Science in Sports and Exercise:* June 2010. Volume 42, Issue 6. Pages 1162-1173. doi: 10.1249/MSS.0b013e3181c74e38

[210] Stout, J.; Cramer, J.; Mielke, M.; et al. "Effects of Twenty-Eight Days of Beta-Alanine and Creatine Monohydrate Supplementation on the Physical Working Capacity at Neuromuscular Fatigue Threshold". *Journal of Strength and Conditioning Research:* November 2006. Volume 20, Issue 4. Pages 928-931. doi: 10.1519/R-19655.1

[211] Kern, B.; Robinson, T. "Effects of Beta-Alanine supplementation on performance and body composition in collegiate wrestlers and football players". *Journal of Strength and Conditioning Research:* July 2011. Volume 25, Issue 7. Pages 1804-1815. doi: 10.1519/JSC.0b013e3181e741cf

[212] Bellinger, P.; Minahan, C. "The effect of β-alanine supplementation on cycling time trials of different length". *European Journal of Sport Science:* December 2015. Pages 829-836. doi: 10.1080/17461391.2015.1120782

[213] Platell, C.; Kong, S.; McCauley, R.; et al. "Branched-chain amino acids". *Journal of Gastroenterology and Hepatology:* July 2000. Volume 15, Issue 7. Pages 706-717. doi: 10.1046/j.1440-1746.2000.02205.x

[214] Norton, L.; Layman, D. "Leucine Regulates Translation Initiation of Protein Synthesis in Skeletal Muscle After Exercise". *Journal of Nutrition:* February 2006. Pages 533S-537S. doi: 10.1093/jn/136.2.533S

[215] Jacobsen, L. (March 19, 2013). Five Intra-Workout Supplements. Retrieved from FitnessRXforWomen: https://www.fitnessrxwomen.com/nutrition/supplements/five-intra-workout-supplements/

[216] MacLean, D.; Graham, T.; Saltin, B. "Branched-chain amino acids augment ammonia metabolism while attenuating protein breakdown during exercise". *American Journal of Physiology, Endocrinology, and Metabolism:* December 1994. Volume 267, Issue 6. Pages E1010-E1022. doi: 10.1152/ajpendo.1994.267.6.E1010

[217] Blomstrand, E.; Eliasson, J.; Karlsson, H.; Köhnke, R. "Branched-Chain Amino Acids Activate Key Enzymes in Protein Synthesis after Physical Exercise". *The Journal of Nutrition:* January 2006. Volume 136, Issue 1. Pages 269S-273S. doi: 10.1093/jn/136.1.269S

[218] Sharp, C.; Pearson, D. "Amino Acid Supplements and Recovery from High-Intensity Resistance Training". *Journal of Strength and Conditioning Research:* April 2010. Volume 24, Issue 4. Pages 1125-1130. doi: 10.1519/JSC.0b013e3181c7c655

[219] Shimomura, Y.; Yamamoto, Y.; Bjotoo, G.; et al. "Neutraceutical Effects of Branched-Chain Amino Acids on Skeletal Muscle". *Journal of Nutrition:* February 2006. Volume 136, Issue 2. Pages 529S-532S. doi: 10.1093/jn/136.2.529S

[220] Nosaka, K.; Sacco, P.; Mawatari, K. "Effects of Amino Acid Supplementation on Muscle Soreness and Damage". *International Journal of Sport Nutrition and Exercise Metabolism:* December 2006. Volume 16, Issue 6. Pages 620-635. doi: 10.1123/ijsnem.16.6.620

[221] Andrews, B.; Cornell, J. (n.d.) *Telomere Lengthening: Curing all diseases including cancer and aging.* Reno, NV: Sierra Sciences, LLC.

[222] Healthspan. (n.d.). Healthspan. Retrieved from Dictionary.com: http://www.dictionary.com/browse/healthspan?s=t

[223] Progeria (n.d.). Progeria. Retrieved from Dictionary.com: http://www.dictionary.com/browse/progeria?s=t

[224] Paddock, C. (August 1, 2017). Scientists rejuvenate aging cells from children with progeria. Retrieved from MedicalNewsToday.com: https://www.medicalnewstoday.com/articles/318740.php

[225] Sarkar, P.; Shinton, R. "Hutchison-Guilford progeria syndrome". *Postgraduate Medical Journal:* 2001. Volume 77, Issue 907. Pages 312-317. doi: 10.1136/pmj.77.907.312

[226] Fossel, Michael. The Immortality Edge: Realize the Secrets of Your Telomeres for a Longer, Healthier Life (p. 12). Wiley. Kindle Edition.

[227] Saßenroth, D.; Meyer, A.; Salewsky, B.; et al. "Sports and Exercise at Different Ages and Leukocyte Telomere Length in Later Life – Data from the Berlin Aging Study II (BASE-II)". PLoS One: December 2015. Volume 10, Issue 12. doi: 10.1371/journal.pone.0142131

[228] Laine, M.; Eriksson, J.; Kujala. U. et al. "Effect of Intensive Exercise in Early Adult Life on Telomere Length in Later Life in Men". *Journal of Sports Science and Medicine:* May 2015. Volume 14, Issue 2. Pages 239-245.

[229] Puterman, E.; Lin, J.; Blackburn, E. "The Power of Exercise: Buffering the Effect of Chronic Stress on Telomere Length". *PLoS One:* May 2010. Volume 5, Issue 5. doi: 10.1371/journal.pone.0010837

230 General Physical Activities Defined by Level of Intensity. (n.d.) General Physical Activities Defined by Level of Intensity. Retrieved from CDC.gov: https://www.cdc.gov/nccdphp/dnpa/physical/pdf/pa_intensity_table_2_1.pdf

231 Cherkas, L.; Hunkin, J.; Kato, B.; et al. "The Association Between Physical Activity in Leisure Time and Leukocyte Telomere Length". *Archives of Internal Medicine:* January 2008. Volume 168, Issue 2. Pages 154-158. doi: 10.1001/archinternmed.2007.3

232 Ogawa, E.; Leveille, S.; Wright, J.; et al. "Physical Activity Domains/Recommendations and Leukocyte Telomere Length in US Adults". *Medicine and Science in Sports and Exercise:* March 2017. Volume 49, Issue 7. Pages 1375-1382. doi: 10.1249/MSS.0000000000001253

233 Body Measurements. (n.d.) Body Measurements. Retrieved from US Centers for Disease Control: https://www.cdc.gov/nchs/fastats/body-measurements.htm

234 Ruiz-Núñez, B.; Pruimboom, L.; Dijck-Brouwer, J.; et al. "Lifestyle and nutritional imbalances associated with Western diseases: causes and consequences of chronic systemic low-grade inflammation in an evolutionary context". *The Journal of Biochemistry:* July 2013. Volume 24, Issue 7. Pages 1183-1201. doi: 10.1016/j.jnutbio.2013.02.009

235 Palahniuk, Chuck. *Fight Club: A Novel* (p. 46). W. W. Norton & Company. Kindle Edition.

236 Moore, S.; Patel, A.; Matthews, C. et al. "Leisure Time Physical Activity of Moderate to Vigorous Intensity and Mortality: A Large Pooled Cohort Analysis". *PLOS Medicine:* November 2012. Volume 9, Issue 11. Pages 1-14. doi: 10.1371/journal.pmed.1001335

237 Darling, M.; Men's Health Editors. (October 6, 2016). How an Out-Of-Shape Air Force Pilot Shed His Spare Tire. Retrieved from Men's Health: https://www.menshealth.com/guy-wisdom/mens-health-ultimate-guy-finalist-otis-hooper

238 Want to Become a Pro Bodybuilder? Here's How. (n.d.) Want to Become a Pro Bodybuilder? Here's How. Retrieved from Generation Iron Fitness Network: https://generationiron.com/want-become-pro-bodybuilder-heres/

239 Mr and Ms Olympia. (n.d.) Mr and Ms Olympia. Retrieved from BodyBuild.com: http://www.bodybuildbid.com/articles/mrolympia/olympqualify.html

Made in the USA
Lexington, KY
20 October 2018